Cancer Etiology, Diagnosis and Treatments

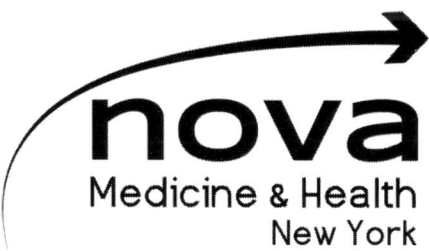

Cancer Etiology, Diagnosis and Treatments

Acute Myeloid Leukemia: Diagnosis, Prognosis, Treatment and Outcomes
Rina Kansal, M.D. (Editor)
2024. ISBN: 979-8-89113-299-3 (Hardcover)
2024. ISBN: 979-8-89113-385-3 (eBook)

Current Therapeutic Strategies for the Management of Cancer
Priyanka Kriplani, PhD (Editor)
Ashwani Kumar Dhingra, PhD (Editor)
Ajmer Singh Grewal, PhD (Editor)
Geeta Deswal, PhD (Editor)
Bhawna Chopra, PhD (Editor)
Peeyush Kaushik (Editor)
2023. ISBN: 979-8-89113-133-0 (Hardcover)
2023. ISBN: 979-8-89113-197-2 (eBook)

Platinum-Based Chemotherapy: Clinical Uses, Efficacy and Side Effects
Kulmira Nurgali, PhD (Editor)
Raquel Abalo Delgado, PhD (Editor)
2022. ISBN: 978-1-68507-972-7 (Hardcover)
2022. ISBN: 979-8-88697-262-7 (eBook)

How Plant Flavonoids Affect the Outcome of Hormonal and Biological Cancer Therapies: A Handbook for Doctors and Patients
Katrin Sak, PhD (Editor)
2022. ISBN: 978-1-68507-608-5 (Hardcover)
2022. ISBN: 978-1-68507-698-6 (eBook)

More information about this series can be found at
https://novapublishers.com/product-category/series/cancer-etiology-diagnosis-and-treatments/

Arli Aditya Parikesit
Editor

A Closer Look at Cancer Biomarkers

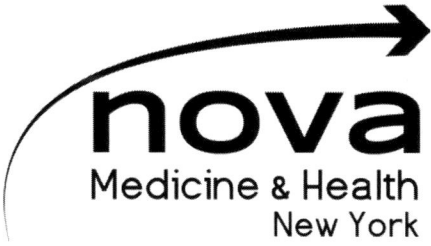

Copyright © 2024 by Nova Science Publishers, Inc.

All rights reserved. No part of this book may be reproduced, stored in a retrieval system or transmitted in any form or by any means: electronic, electrostatic, magnetic, tape, mechanical photocopying, recording or otherwise without the written permission of the Publisher.

We have partnered with Copyright Clearance Center to make it easy for you to obtain permissions to reuse content from this publication. Please visit copyright.com and search by Title, ISBN, or ISSN.

For further questions about using the service on copyright.com, please contact:

Copyright Clearance Center
Phone: +1-(978) 750-8400   Fax: +1-(978) 750-4470   E-mail: info@copyright.com

NOTICE TO THE READER

The Publisher has taken reasonable care in the preparation of this book but makes no expressed or implied warranty of any kind and assumes no responsibility for any errors or omissions. No liability is assumed for incidental or consequential damages in connection with or arising out of information contained in this book. The Publisher shall not be liable for any special, consequential, or exemplary damages resulting, in whole or in part, from the readers' use of, or reliance upon, this material. Any parts of this book based on government reports are so indicated and copyright is claimed for those parts to the extent applicable to compilations of such works.

Independent verification should be sought for any data, advice or recommendations contained in this book. In addition, no responsibility is assumed by the Publisher for any injury and/or damage to persons or property arising from any methods, products, instructions, ideas or otherwise contained in this publication.

This publication is designed to provide accurate and authoritative information with regards to the subject matter covered herein. It is sold with the clear understanding that the Publisher is not engaged in rendering legal or any other professional services. If legal or any other expert assistance is required, the services of a competent person should be sought. FROM A DECLARATION OF PARTICIPANTS JOINTLY ADOPTED BY A COMMITTEE OF THE AMERICAN BAR ASSOCIATION AND A COMMITTEE OF PUBLISHERS.

Library of Congress Cataloging-in-Publication Data

ISBN: 979-8-89113-497-3

Published by Nova Science Publishers, Inc. † New York

Dedication

This book is dedicated to all the cancer patients, survivors, and caregivers who have bravely faced this disease and shared their stories with us. Their courage and resilience have motivated us to pursue our research and education in cancer biomarkers, with the hope of finding better ways to prevent, diagnose, and treat cancer.

We also dedicate this book to our mentors, colleagues, and students who have contributed to the advancement of canceromics as a multidisciplinary field that integrates genomics, proteomics, metabolomics, and bioinformatics. Their passion and creativity have enriched our knowledge and understanding of cancer biology and medicine.

Finally, we dedicate this book to our families and friends who have supported us throughout our careers and lives. Their love and encouragement have given us the strength and joy to continue our work and fulfill our mission.

Contents

Foreword		ix
Preface		xi
Acknowledgment		xiii
Chapter 1	**Structural Bioinformatics Approach in Carcinogenesis** ....1 Nausheen Bhat, Raechell Raechell, Ryan Widjaja and Arli Aditya Parikesit	
Chapter 2	**In Silico Design of a Novel Multi-Epitope Peptide Cancer Vaccine against Non-Small Cell Lung Cancer (NSCLC) for the Indonesian Population** ....7 Tiffanny Adora Putri, Felicia Edgina Susilo, Stanly Dewanto, Vivi Julietta, Axel F. Shiloputra and Arli Aditya Parikesit	
Chapter 3	**The Molecular Docking Approach toward Targeting Transcription Factors in Prostate Cancer** ....29 Aileen Gunawan, Joan Nadia and Arli Aditya Parikesit	
Chapter 4	**A Closer Look at Cancer Biomarkers: Their Updated Uses for the Diagnosis and Treatment of Cancer** ....39 Carlos A. González Núñez, Daniel A. García Padilla and Alberto Monroy Chargoy	

Chapter 5	**Classification and Identification of Gene Markers in the Medulloblastoma Subgroup by Implementing the Support Vector Machine 53**
	Lalu Bayu Dwi Cahyo and Rohmatul Fajriyah
Chapter 6	**Prostate Cancer Biomarkers 69**
	Maxim N. Peshkov and Igor V. Reshetov
Chapter 7	**Tissue Markers of Prostate Cancer (Review) 91**
	Maxim N. Peshkov and Igor V. Reshetov
Chapter 8	**Serum Markers of Prostate Cancer (A Review) 119**
	Maxim N. Peshkov and Igor V. Reshetov

About the Editor 137

Index 139

Foreword

Cancer is a complex and heterogeneous disease that affects millions of people worldwide. Despite the advances in diagnosis and treatment, many challenges remain in the fight against cancer. One of the most promising areas of research is the identification and validation of cancer biomarkers, which are molecules or characteristics that can indicate the presence, progression, or response to therapy of cancer. Cancer biomarkers can provide valuable information for clinicians and patients, such as early detection, prognosis, risk stratification, and personalized treatment. However, the discovery and development of cancer biomarkers is not a straightforward process. It requires rigorous methods, multidisciplinary collaboration, and careful evaluation of the clinical utility and impact of each biomarker.

This book aims to provide a comprehensive and updated overview of the current state and future directions of cancer biomarker research. It covers various aspects of cancer biomarker discovery, validation, and clinical implementation, as well as the challenges and opportunities in this field. The book also showcases some of the most recent and innovative applications of cancer biomarkers in various types of cancers, such as breast, lung, colorectal, prostate, ovarian, and pancreatic cancer. The book is intended for researchers, clinicians, students, and anyone who is interested in learning more about the potential and limitations of cancer biomarkers.

Arli Aditya Parikesit
Editor

Preface

Cancer is a complex and heterogeneous disease that poses significant challenges for diagnosis, prognosis, and treatment. In recent years, advances in molecular biology and biotechnology have enabled the discovery and development of various biomarkers that can provide valuable information about cancer. Biomarkers are substances or processes that indicate the presence or state of cancer in the body. They can be derived from the tumor itself or from the host response to the tumor. They can be measured in different types of samples, such as blood, tissue, urine, or saliva. They can also be detected by different methods, such as genomic, epigenomic, proteomic, glycomic, or imaging techniques. Biomarkers have multiple applications in cancer research and medicine. They can be used to assess the risk of developing cancer, to diagnose cancer at an early stage, to predict the prognosis and response to treatment of cancer patients, to monitor the effectiveness and toxicity of therapy, and to detect the recurrence or progression of cancer. Biomarkers can also facilitate the development of new drugs and therapies by identifying potential targets and surrogate endpoints. Biomarkers can also enable personalized medicine by matching the right treatment to the right patient based on their molecular profile.

This book aims to provide a comprehensive overview of the current state of the art and future perspectives of cancer biomarkers. It covers the basic concepts and definitions of biomarkers, their role and utility in cancer research and medicine, their types and sources, their detection methods and technologies, their validation criteria and strategies, their clinical applications and implications, their challenges and limitations. It also presents some examples of successful biomarker discovery and development in various types of cancer. Chapter 1 provides a solid background on structural bioinformatics approach in carcinogenesis. It also elicits the important role of bioinformatics in the annotation of cancer biomarkers. Chapter 2 provides immunoinformatics method to design non-small cell lung cancer for Indonesian population. It provides computational tools for standard vaccine design of Cancer. Thus, chapter 3 provides more insight on molecular docking approach for designing prostate cancer lead compounds. It showcases the importance of molecular simulation in rational drug design for cancer therapy. Chapter 4 is focusing on diagnosis and treatment of cancer, along with it's possible clinical setting. Chapter 5 is introducing the application of support vector macine in the identification of gene marker. It elicited R-based pipeline that should be reproducible and easy-to use for any bioinformaticians. Lastly, chapter 6 is focusing on multifacets of prostate cancer biomarkers.

The book is intended for a broad audience of researchers, clinicians, students, policy makers, industry representatives, patients, advocates, and anyone interested in learning more about cancer biomarkers. It is written by experts in the field who share their knowledge and experience with clarity and rigor. We hope that this book will serve as a useful resource and reference for anyone who wants to gain a deeper understanding of cancer biomarkers and their potential impact on cancer prevention, detection, diagnosis, prognosis, treatment, monitoring, recurrence, research, development, innovation, personalization, ethics, and society. The editor would like to thanks to Department of Research and Community Service of Indonesia International Institute for Life Sciences (i3L) for supporting this initiative.

Arli Aditya Parikesit,
Associate Professor, Dr.,
Indonesia International Institute for Life Sciences, Indonesia

Acknowledgment

The editor would like to thank Nova publisher for facilitating the publication of this book. Moreover, thanks also go to the Innovation and Entrepreneurship Department of Indonesia International Institute for Life Sciences, for their heartfelt support. Many thanks also to the authors of the book chapters for contributing their great intellectual works in cancer biomarker. Lastly, many thanks to Indonesian Society of Bioinformatics and Biodiversity (ISBB) for initiating national discussion and discourse on canceromics and cancer informatics.

Chapter 1

Structural Bioinformatics Approach in Carcinogenesis

Nausheen Bhat
Raechell Raechell
Ryan Widjaja
and Arli Aditya Parikesit[*]
Department of Bioinformatics, School of Life Sciences, Indonesia International Institute for Life Sciences, Jakarta, Indonesia

Abstract

Cancer remains a prevalent disease with no specific treatments. Advances in structural bioinformatics have benefited a variety of fields in modern biology, particularly biomedical practices for drug design. From advancements in information technology to developing tools that screen for genetic expressions, structural bioinformatics has much more to offer in cancer research than in the last two decades. The presence of mutations and their comparisons to normal genes and proteins shed light on how cancer develops, and the crystallization of these proteins aids in understanding the cause of mutation. The article examines whether structural bioinformatics practices can benefit cancer research, the tools used, and how to expand the subject.

Keywords: structural bioinformatics, cancer, tumor, protein, genetic expression

---

[*] Corresponding Author's Email: arli.parikesit@i3l.ac.id.

In: A Closer Look at Cancer Biomarkers
Editor: Arli Aditya Parikesit
ISBN: 979-8-89113-497-3
© 2024 Nova Science Publishers, Inc.

Introduction

Biological research has seen many advancements and is a growing, dynamic field. One of the significant developments in modern biology is the application of bioinformatics to medical practices. Bioinformatics has influenced and pushed the boundaries of modern biology, from computer programs and biological algorithms to pertinent databanks and impeccable software (Chou, 2004). Bioinformatics has provided headway for protein sciences through structural bioinformatics, circumventing most complications due to its dynamic principles (Gail et al., 2003).

Structural Bioinformatics is the specific study of analyzing and predicting the third-dimensional structure of proteins, along with Deoxyribose nucleic acid (DNA) and Ribose nucleic acid (RNA). Structural bioinformatics' approaches in protein have been in creating renowned databases and portals, such as SWISS-PROT, GenProtEC, and ExPASy, that cover gene ontologies of organisms and their proteins produced (Gail et al., 2003). The protein information obtained through structural bioinformatics is its basic structure, the protein–ligand complexes, enzyme classifications, and most importantly, protein structure–function relations. In the field of biomedical research, structural bioinformatics has pioneered drug discovery and drug design. Designing drugs has become much easier due to the tools present due to technological advancements. Due to protein motif databanks such as PROSITE, developments in high-throughput crystallography and Nuclear Magnetic Resonance (NMR), designing and identifying drugs has become much more accessible, and therefore, more implemented bioinformatics methodologies in the steps to analyzing drugs (Tom et al., 2006).

Even though there has been significant progress in technology and its biological applications, structural bioinformatics still has much more to offer in cancer studies. Structural bioinformatics, with all its abilities in gene predictions and protein interactions, has only scratched the surface of canceromics. It is a specialized study regarding cancer production, proliferation, and metastasis and with the genes and gene interactions involved. In this article, we will discuss the implementation of structural bioinformatics and its use against cancer in general and, more specifically, breast, colon, and lung cancer.

Material and Methods

The utilization of specific tools in structural bioinformatics process pipelines such as screening, analysis, and predictions. Some of these materials are as follows:

Biomarkers

Biomarkers have been a critical factor in the identification of cancer. Research has shown that implementing specialized biomarkers with accurate results in scenarios where specific screening procedures did not show predicted outcomes (Jinong Li, 2002). The biomarkers also provide screening that can detect early stages of cancers. Structural bioinformatics can play a large part in identifying suitable biomarkers for cancer. Specific proteins for cancer biomarkers should proceed with mass spectrometry, microarrays, and protein–reading–specific software (Jinong Li, 2002).

Microarray

To better understand cancers, it is essential to analyze the molecular levels of the cancer. As mentioned, biomarkers can represent the diagnosis on a molecular level, but in some cases, these biomarkers may need more help due to the few tumour markers. However, by reading the genetic expressions of the cancer cells, a proper diagnosis can be determined. Regardless, microarray still has similar constraints to biomarkers in that it would be less effective if the sample sizes were small (Kim, 2004).

Protein Databanks

With the development of information technology, databases have become more interactive and provide several different forms of data collected through laboratory methods. In today's time, specific cancer-related proteins have been crystallized and can be accessed through these databases, along with this sequence and other information, ready to be analyzed. Crystallography has been a crucial part of protein biology and has now provided more leeway into cancer research as information regarding the function and three-dimensional structures of these protein crystals can be publicly available within online databases. Identification of mutation within normal genes is a very complex and meticulous procedure. To sum it up conveniently, it is as follows the step-by-step process of identifying cancer mutations from genes.

The first step requires the understanding of the genetic sequence. From the sequences alone, we can identify the mutational differences. We then screen the two samples in a microarray with different fluorescent markers. Another use of the bioinformatics tool would be the data collection, where the data is produced by the microarray and collected. The data would record the intensity of the mutations and replications of the different genes within a gene region. These replications can be identified based on the fluorescence colour, where, in this case, red represents high intensity and green represents low intensity. Depending on the intensity level, anything in between would be a dimmer shade of either colour.

Result and Discussion

Crystallography also plays a vital role since it can identify mutations, even when the result is cancer. The mutations in a region of the BRCA1 gene, identified as the BRCT region, can mutate to disallow tumour suppression and, therefore, cause increasing growth of breast cancer (R. et al., 2001). These crucial mutations define the growth and proliferation of cancers, especially breast cancer, one of the most common types of cancer. Although Crystallography does not cure the mutation or act as a treatment, it provides insight into approaching these mutating protein regions and better understanding the mutations for further research.

Furthermore, understanding the protein interactions between cancer-related proteins express the differences between regular and mutated proteins (Gozde Kar, 2009). The function–mutation relationship of specific proteins can also be analyzed, where the p53 tumour suppressor protein was subject to mutation and then compared to identify the structure–function and function–mutation changes within the protein (Shunsuke Kato, 2003). The shown result is as a form of a heatmap, where 2314 missense mutants of p53 plus p53. Each column represents a p53 mutant, whereas each row represents a p53 promoter—the difference between the mutation and the identified promoter with the fluorescence.

Structural bioinformatics still has an interesting technique that can pursue the outcome of breast cancer. Structural bioinformatics also deals with the dynamic state of proteins. It provides insight into where the mutation may occur based on the current structure and, more importantly, the protein's function (Ian W Taylor1, 2009).

The bioinformatics concepts of systems biology could identify the specific genes in the progressive states, where each gene can represent the level of regulation in patients. Similar to the clusters, it is colour-coded based on the intensity of correlation in prognosis patients (Ian W Taylor1, 2009). This network also shows the relations between the cancer–related genes and how they may influence one another considering the occurrence of mutation.

Conclusion

Understanding proteins' structural and functional impacts to identify diseases has many benefits. Structural bioinformatics has provided several tools for developing protein sciences, drug design, and drug discovery. However, even though by implementing all these tools for cancer research and treatments, there are only some provided benefits of structural bioinformatics. With the implementation of structural bioinformatics, cancer research now better understands the genetic and protein–based information that can influence cancer growth. Several techniques and tools, as mentioned, can benefit in accurately reading and identifying cancer growth. Biomarkers and microarrays are fine tools that can be used for analysis, whereas protein databanks can assist in understanding better the functional errors caused during cancer growth.

However, there is a lack of research based on the practical use of structural bioinformatics that can help prevent cancer and counter it before the later stages.

Therefore, more research should proceed to implement bioinformatics techniques into cancer–based medical practices.

Acknowledgments

We thank the Research Institute and Community Service (LPPM) of Indonesia International Institute for Life Sciences for the opportunity to develop this research article. Moreover, thanks also go to the Community Language Center of Indonesia International Institute for Life Sciences for their excellent proofreading of our manuscript.

References

Bartlett G. J., Todd A. E., Thornton J. M. (2003). Inferring Protein Function From Structure. *Structural Bioinformatics*.

Blundell T. L., Sibanda B. L., Montalvão R. W., Brewerton S., Chelliah V., Worth C. L., Harmer N. J., Davies O., and Burke D. (2006). Structural biology and bioinformatics in drug design: opportunities and challenges for target identification and lead discovery. *Philosophical Transactions of the Royal Society*, 413 - 423.

Chou, K.-C. (2004). Structural Bioinformatics and its Impact on Biomedical Science. *Current Medicinal Chemistry*, pp. 2105–2134.

Kato S., Han S. Y., Liu W., Otsuka K., Shibata H., Kanamaru R., and Ishioka C. (2003). Understanding the function–structure and function– mutation relationships of p53 tumour suppressor protein by high-resolution missense mutation analysis. *PNAS*, 8424–8429.

Kar G., Gursoy A., Keskin O. (2009). Human Cancer Protein-Protein Interaction Network: A Structural Perspective. *PLoS Computational Biology*.

Kim, H. (2004). Role of Microarray in Cancer Diagnosis. *Cancer Research and Treatment*.

Li J., Zhang Z., Rosenzweig J., Wang Y. Y., and Chan D. W. (2002). Proteomics and Bioinformatics Approaches for Identification of Serum Biomarkers to Detect Breast Cancer. *Clinical Chemistry*, 1296 - 1304.

Taylor I. W., Linding R., Warde-Farley D., Liu Y., Pesquita C., Faria D., Bull S., Pawson T., Morris Q., & Wrana J. L.. (2009). Dynamic modularity in protein interaction networks predicts breast cancer outcome. *Nature Biotechnology*.

Williams R. S., Green R., and Glover J. N. (2001). Crystal structure of the BRCT repeat region from the breast cancer-associated protein BRCA1. *Nature Structural Biology*.

Chapter 2

In Silico Design of a Novel Multi-Epitope Peptide Cancer Vaccine against Non-Small Cell Lung Cancer (NSCLC) for the Indonesian Population

Tiffanny Adora Putri[1]
Felicia Edgina Susilo[1]
Stanly Dewanto[1]
Vivi Julietta[1]
Axel F. Shiloputra[2]
and Arli Aditya Parikesit[2,*]

[1]Department of Biomedicine, Indonesia International Institute for Life Sciences, Jakarta, Indonesia
[2]Department of Bioinformatics, School of Life Sciences, Indonesia International Institute for Life Sciences, Jakarta, Indonesia

Abstract

The main reason for pursuing this research was because lung cancer continues to be the most significant cause of cancer-related death worldwide. Thankfully, identifying several genes crucial to cancer development has resulted in the development of targeted therapies like cancer vaccines shown to increase the specificity of treatment for afflicted cells and increase survival rates. Consequently, this work aims to develop an immunoinformatics-based multi-epitope peptide cancer

---

* Corresponding Author's Email: arli.parikesit@i3l.ac.id.

In: A Closer Look at Cancer Biomarkers
Editor: Arli Aditya Parikesit
ISBN: 979-8-89113-497-3
© 2024 Nova Science Publishers, Inc.

vaccine against NSCLC for the Indonesian population. Before developing a vaccine, CTL, HTL, and B-cell epitopes were predicted and evaluated for their population coverage. After creating the vaccine, it will examine its physicochemical, allergenic, and antigenic qualities. Various bioinformatics techniques will model, validate, and dock the construct. The proposed vaccine architecture can reach 95.47 per cent of Indonesians, has good physicochemical and antigenic qualities, and is considered non-allergenic. The BPIFA1 antigen, which targets explicitly particular HLA alleles seen in the Indonesian population, was successfully used in this investigation to identify and create a possible NSCLC cancer vaccine.

Keywords: NSCLC, vaccine, epitopes, BPIFA1, HLA, Indonesia

Introduction

Lung cancer is the leading cause of cancer-related mortality around the world. Non-small cell lung cancer causes around 85% of lung cancer [1]. malignant cells formed in the lung tissues cause Non-small cell lung cancer (NSCLC) when a healthy cell starts to go out of control and forms a tumour. There are three types of NSCLC, including squamous cell carcinoma, large cell carcinoma, and adenocarcinoma [2]. In 2020, there were approximately 2.2 million new lung cancer cases, with 1.8 million deaths related to lung cancer. This number represents about 10% of all new cancer cases and 20% of all cancer deaths in 2020 [3]. However, this number is much smaller in Indonesia at approximately 8.6% and 12.6% respectively [4]. In addition, the lung cancer incidence rate in Indonesia is 19.4 in 100,000 people, with a mortality rate of 10.9 in 100,000 people [5]. Fortunately, because of advances in cancer therapy and treatments, the 2-year and 5-year relative survival of NSCLC has rapidly increased to 42% and 21.7% in the last decade.

Various treatments have been developed to eliminate NSCLC. Cancer treatment uses standard methods such as surgery, chemotherapy, and radiotherapy. Unfortunately, chemotherapy needs to be accompanied by primary supportive care, and it is known to be able to reduce the quality of life. Aside from that, adverse events may also arise either during or after the chemotherapy process. Meanwhile, radiotherapy also provides another solution as a cancer treatment, although it showed poor survival and low local control [6]. Recently, due to the discovery of several genes that are intensely involved in the progression of cancer, the emergence of targeted therapy has been studied further to improve the survival rate and quality of life by increasing the specificity of the therapy toward the affected cells. One of the most common targeted therapies is immunotherapy, specifically cancer vaccines. Cancer vaccines trigger the immune system by priming using the cancer-related antigen to target the related cancer cells. Cancer vaccines offer a specific treatment for eradicating the tumour, which leads to decreased cytotoxicity towards the normal healthy cells [7-8]. Among others, peptide-based vaccines are promising in triggering immune responses against cancer cells [9]. A vaccine composed of several peptides, called multi-epitope vaccines, is stated to be ideal and practical since it induces broader immune responses [10-11]. Multi-epitope vaccines may cover a broader population and exclude adverse reactions [12].

Recent advancement in bioinformatics tools reportedly plays a part in easing the development of multi-epitope vaccines [13]. The immunoinformatics approaches significantly help increase efficiency, reducing time, money, and effort compared to the conventional method [14]. The *in-silico* approaches, for instance, allow the identification of suitable epitopes, which remain the major challenge in cancer immunotherapy [15]. Moreover, it also aids in the prediction and analysis of epitopes that can stimulate both CD4+ helper T lymphocytes (HTL) and CD8+ cytotoxic T lymphocytes (CTL) responses, which reportedly are essential qualities of an efficient cancer vaccine [16]. Various widely available tools help in many stages of development, starting from identification, design, prediction, and analysis. Considering everything, this study aims to utilize immunoinformatics methods in designing a multi-epitope peptide cancer vaccine against NSCLC for the Indonesian population.

Material and Methods

Cancer Antigen Selection

The cancer antigen used is the lung-specific X protein (LunX) BPIFA1. This protein shows high expression on NSCLC cells but no expression on normal human lung tissues or other tissues from the major organs.

Sequence Retrieval

The UniProt database (https://www.uniprot.org/) retrieved the canonical amino acid sequence of BPIFA1 (UniProt ID: Q9NP55). The specific HLA allele sequences that can match with the select epitopes were retrieved, and the granulocyte-macrophage colony-stimulating factor (GM-CSF) (UniProt ID: P04141) sequence was retrieved as an adjuvant.

HLA Allele Identification

In order to find out the HLA alleles of the Indonesian population, a search through 'The Allele Frequency Net Database (http://allelefrequencies.net/), specifically the 'HLA Classical Allele Freq Search' was conducted. The parameters that were adjusted were "Indonesia" in the country tab. For the selection, HLA class I A and B and class II DRB1 alleles with more than 5% frequencies were chosen for further generation and analysis of peptides.

MHC Class I Peptide Binding and Immunogenicity Prediction

Prediction of the peptides binding to cytotoxic T-cells (CTLs) used netCTLpan (https://services.healthtech.dtu.dk/service.php?NetCTLpan-1.1). The BPIFA1 amino acid sequence was posted on the sequence column of netCTLpan, and the previously chosen HLA class I A and B alleles were selected. The parameters for peptide length, threshold for showing predictions, weight on C terminal cleavage, weight on TAP transport efficiency, and threshold for epitope identification were defaulted. Meanwhile, the prediction was sorted by the combined Score. The peptide epitopes denoted by the E-value were selected as they fall under the 1% threshold. The immunogenicity of the selected peptide epitopes of BPIFA1 was then analyzed using IEDB (http://tools.iedb.org/immunogenicity/). The peptide sequences were immediately pasted and submitted without changing any parameters. A positive immunogenicity score indicates that the peptide is immunogenic.

MHC Class II Peptide Binding Prediction

Prediction of the peptide binding to MHC Class II was conducted using netMHCII-pan 4.0 (https://services.healthtech.dtu.dk/service.php?NetMHCII

pan-4.0). Both protein sequences of BPIFA1 and HLA-DRB1 alleles identified previously inputted accordingly. The peptide length was adjusted for 15, and the strong and weak binding threshold was set to 2% and 10%, respectively. For the selection, peptides that exhibited strong binding were chosen. Following the 15-mer peptide generation, the epitopes were further analyzed for their ability to induce the IFN gamma using IFNepitope tools (http://crdd.osdd.net/raghava/ifnepitope/predict.php). After inserting the peptides, the prediction method set for 'Motif and SVM hybrid,' and the prediction model set for 'IFN-gamma vs. Non-IFN-gamma.' An epitope with a positive SVM score and MERCI score ≥1 preferred the selection.

Antibody Binding Prediction
Further analysis of peptide binding with B-cells was performed through the IEDB Antibody Epitope Prediction (http://tools.iedb.org/bcell/) tools. The antigen sequences were inserted and analyzed using The 'Bepipred Linear Epitope Prediction 2.0' method. The results are selected based on the threshold above 0.5 and the peptide chain with the optimal length.

Population Coverage Analysis
The population coverage of the selected epitope specific to the Indonesian population was determined with the predicted sequences corresponding to the selected HLA alleles, which will be submitted to the IEDB population coverage analysis tool (http://tools.iedb.org/population/). Indonesia area was selected, and class I and II combined were selected as the calculation option. The previously predicted epitopes with their corresponding HLA alleles were then submitted. The tool will compromise the average number of epitopes recognized by the population and the minimum number recognized by 90% of populations.

Vaccine Construct Design

The multi-epitope vaccine construct was designed using an adjuvant and several linkers to link each generated epitope. The literature review was conducted to determine the suitable adjuvant and linkers for the construct design. GM-CSF was chosen as the adjuvant to be linked to the multi-epitope vaccine. Three different linkers are included in this construct: GPGPG, EAAAK, and AAY. GPGPG was used to link between the epitopes of B lymphocytes and helper T lymphocytes. At the same time, the EAAAK linker linked the adjuvant with the vaccine construct, specifically towards the B-cell epitopes. Meanwhile, all of the CTL epitopes were linked using the AAY linker.

Vaccine Construct Analysis

Several aspects of the generated multi-epitope vaccine construct were analyzed, including its antigenicity, allergenicity, and physicochemical properties. SVMTriP web server [17] was utilized to determine the overall antigenicity of the constructed vaccine with 20 amino acids chosen for the antigenic epitope length. The safety of the vaccine was catered with the construct allergenicity parameter. It was tested using the AllerTOP v.2.0 [18]. The physicochemical properties of the vaccine construct were also analyzed, including the half-life, isoelectric point (Pi), molecular weight, sequence length, grand average of hydropathicity (GRAVY), aliphatic index, and protein stability, using ProtParam Expasy web server [19].

Vaccine Construct Modeling

The generated and analyzed multi-epitope vaccine construct was modelled with the I-TASSER server (https://zhanggroup.org/I-TASSER/) by inputting the designed vaccine sequence into the system. The web server predicts the peptide structure through *de novo* peptide structure prediction. The advanced parameters were not changed for this experiment.

Validation of the Vaccine Model

The vaccine model was validated using SWISS-MODEL tools structure assessment (https://swissmodel.expasy.org/assess). The assessment outcome includes a QMEAN score to show the consistency of structural features with the sequence based on predictions. Ramachandran plot was also provided as the outcome of the assessment.

Validation of Peptide Cleavage in Vaccine Model

The vaccine amino acid sequences were submitted back to netCTLpan to validate peptide cleavage and binding to their HLA molecules (https://services.healthtech.dtu.dk/service.php?NetCTLpan-1.1) and netMHCII-pan 4.0 for helper T-cells (https://services.healthtech.dtu.dk/service.php?NetMHCIIpan-4.0).

MHC Molecule Modeling

The MHC (HLA) molecule model was obtained from an established database tested in physiological conditions. The database used for all HLA modelling is pHLA3D (https://www.phla3d.com.br/). All relevant HLA proteins were extracted from the database.

Molecular Docking

The molecular docking of the epitope to the HLA molecule was done using the HPEPDOCK web server (http://huanglab.phys.hust.edu.cn/hpepdock/). The web server predicts the binding of the epitope to the HLA molecule and scores the result. Only the top 10 predicted bindings were analyzed and used in this report. All of the parameters provided by the system were not changed. The molecular docking was then visualized using BIOVIA Discovery Studio Visualizer.

Results

Identified HLA Alleles in Indonesia Population

The HLA alleles of the Indonesian population, class I and class II, with frequencies over 5%, were identified and listed in Table 1. A total of 14 HLA class I and 6 HLA class II were identified and used for further prediction and analysis.

Table 1. Identification of HLA allele of Indonesia population with frequencies more than 5%

	HLA
Class I	HLA-A02:01, HLA-A11:01, HLA-A24:02, HLA-A24:07, HLA-A33:03, HLA-A34:01, HLA-B15:02, HLA-B15:13, HLA-B15:21, HLA-B18:01, HLA-B35:05, HLA-B38:02, HLA-B44:03, HLA-B58:01
Class II	DRB1_0701, DRB1_1101, DRB1_1202, DRB1_1501, DRB1_1502, DRB1_1602

T-Cell and B-Cell Epitopes Candidate

Following the prediction of epitopes from NetCTLpan, NetMHCpan, and IEDB antibody binding prediction, epitopes with good antigenicity, IFN score, and ability to bind to multiple HLAs were selected. Table 2 shows a total of three final candidates of CD8+ epitopes, four final candidates of CD4+ epitopes, and one final candidate of B-cell epitope to be included in the vaccine construct, along with their corresponding antigenicity/IFN scores and respective MHC molecules that bind to them.

Table 2. Candidate of CTL, HTL, and B-cell epitopes

	Antigen	Epitope	Residue Number	Antigenicity Score/IFN Score*	MHC
CD8+	BPIFA1	LYVTIPLGI	128	0.18206	HLA-A*24:02, HLA-A*24:07
		ITAEILAVR	158	0.28975	HLA-A*33:03, HLA-A*34:01
		NMLIHGLQF	243	0.11668	HLA-B*15:02
CD4+	BPIFA1	TIPLGIKLQVNTPLV	132	0.32222562	DRB1_1501, DRB1_1502
		IPLGIKLQVNTPLVG	133	0.47528209	DRB1_1501, DRB1_1502, DRB1_1602
		PLGIKLQVNTPLVGA	134	0.47282917	DRB1_1501, DRB1_1502, DRB1_1602
		LGIKLQVNTPLVGAS	135	0.15418407	DRB1_1501
B-cell		GKVTSVIPGLNNI	93		-

*antigenicity score was applied for the CD8+ epitopes, while IFN score was applied for CD4+ epitopes.

Population Coverage of CTL and HTL Epitopes

The estimated Indonesian population coverage for CTL and HTL epitopes set separately is 90.7% and 51.25%, respectively. The CTL and HTL epitopes set were estimated to cover 95.47% of Indonesia's population.

Construction of Multi-Epitope Peptide Vaccine

The construct was arranged from GM-CSF adjuvant (light blue), B-cell epitopes (dark blue), HTL epitopes (light grey), and CTL epitopes (dark grey), respectively. In between, they were linked by EAAAK linkers (green), GPGPG linkers (yellow), and AAY linkers (black), shown in Figure 1.

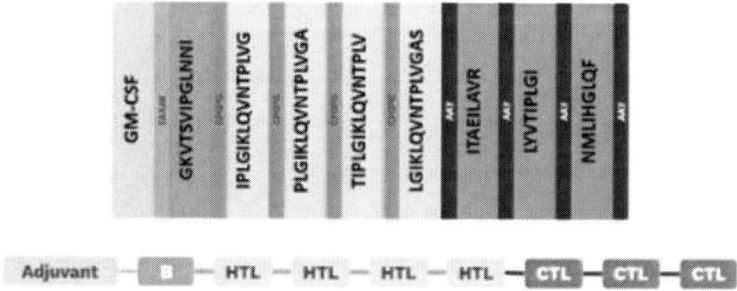

Figure 1. Graphical representation of the multi-epitope vaccine construct. The order from left to right: GM-CSF adjuvant (light blue), EAAAK linker (green), B-cell epitopes (dark blue), GPGPG linkers (yellow), HTL epitopes (light grey), AAY linkers (black), CTL epitopes (dark grey). GM-CSF: granulocyte-macrophage colony-stimulating factors, B: B-cell epitopes, HTL: helper T lymphocyte epitopes, CTL: cytotoxic T lymphocyte epitopes.

Antigenicity, Allergenicity, and Physicochemical Properties of the Multi-Epitope Peptide Vaccine Construct

The vaccine construct is antigenic and non-allergenic, with a sequence length of 281 amino acids. Moreover, the construct has a molecular weight of 29858.89 Da and a theoretical pI 6.89. A stable construct is determined with an instability index below 40, which leads to the conclusion that the construct has suitable stability with an instability index of 39.72. In addition, the half-life of the constructed multi-epitope vaccine was recorded to be 30 hours in mammalian reticulocytes that are maintained *in vitro*, while more than 20 and 10 hours in yeast and *Escherichia coli* in the *in vivo* settings, respectively. The construct also obtained sufficient thermostability, recorded by the high aliphatic index (104.84). Lastly, the grand average hydropathicity (GRAVY) is 0.170, indicating a hydrophobic construct.

Vaccine Construct Modeling

All selected eight epitopes were constructed into a multi-epitope vaccine from 281 amino acids, and the model was predicted and visualized using I-TASSER. The server prediction model resulted in 5 different models, ranging from the worst to the best model. Two of the models were picked from the list, the vaccine model 1 and 5 (Figure 2).

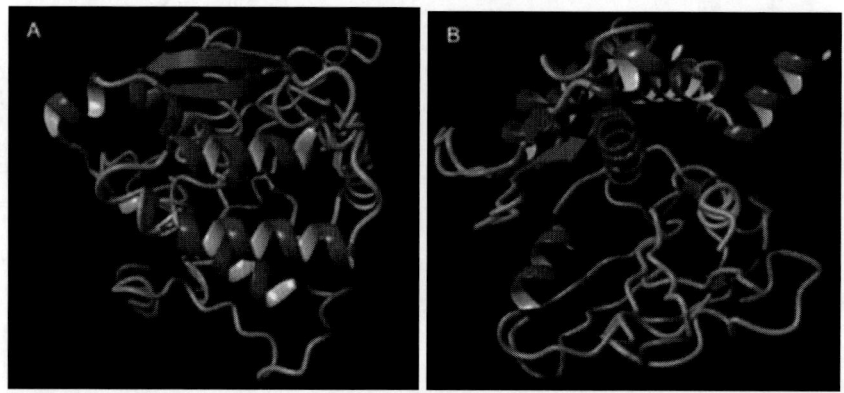

Figure 2. Visual representation of the vaccine constructs using I-TASSER. (A) Predicted vaccine model 1 with a c-score of -3.96, (B) Predicted vaccine model 5 with a c-score of -2.52.

Validation of the Vaccine Model

The vaccine model structure was validated, and the Ramachandran plot was measured (Figure 3). The Ramachandran favoured value for model 1 is 55.88%, while the value for model 5 is 73.88%. Further analysis also shows the qRMSD value for model 1 at 0.44±0.05, model 5 at 0.45±0.05, and MolProbity for model 1 at 4.40 and model 5 at 2.75. Therefore, the predicted vaccine model 5 (Figure 2B) is more favourable structurally than vaccine model 1.

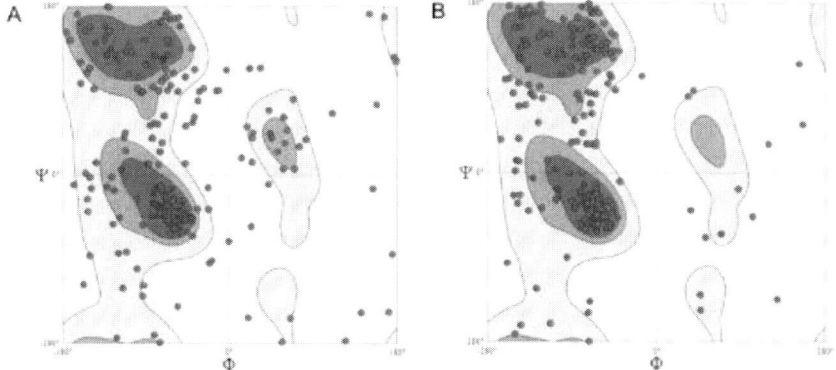

Figure 3. Ramachandran Plot for structure validation of vaccine model. (A) Predicted vaccine model 1 plot, with Ramachandran-favored value at 55.88%, outlier value at 23.53%, qRMSD value at 0.44±0.05, (B) Predicted vaccine model 5 plot, with Ramachandran-favored value at 73.88%, outlier value at 8.96%, qRMSD value at 0.45±0.05.

Validation of Peptide Cleavage in Vaccine Model

In addition to structural validation, peptide cleavage and binding capability were tested using the constructed vaccine model (281 amino acids). The result shows successful cleavage and binding capability to its respective HLA binding partners (Table 3).

Table 3. Validation of peptide cleavage and their binding capability to their HLA binding partners. Identical cleavage means that the peptide sequence is conserved. Binder means that the peptide could bind to the original HLA binding partners, as stated in Table 2

Peptide (Epitope)	Identical Cleavage	Binding Capability
IPLGIKLQVNTPLVG	Yes	Binder
PLGIKLQVNTPLVGA	Yes	Binder
TIPLGIKLQVNTPLV	Yes	Binder
LGIKLQVNTPLVGAS	Yes	Binder
ITAEILAVR	Yes	Binder
LYVTIPLGI	Yes	Binder
NMLIHGLQF	Yes	Binder

MHC Molecule Modeling

The model of the MHC molecule was extracted from the database. A total of 8 MHC molecules were relevant in the study, namely HLA-A*24:02, HLA*24:07, HLA-A*33:03, HLA-A*34:01, HLA-B*15:02, DRB1_15:01, DRB1_15:02, DRB1_16:02. However, HLA-A*24:07 was unavailable in the database. Thus, the authors decided not to include it in the study (Figure 4).

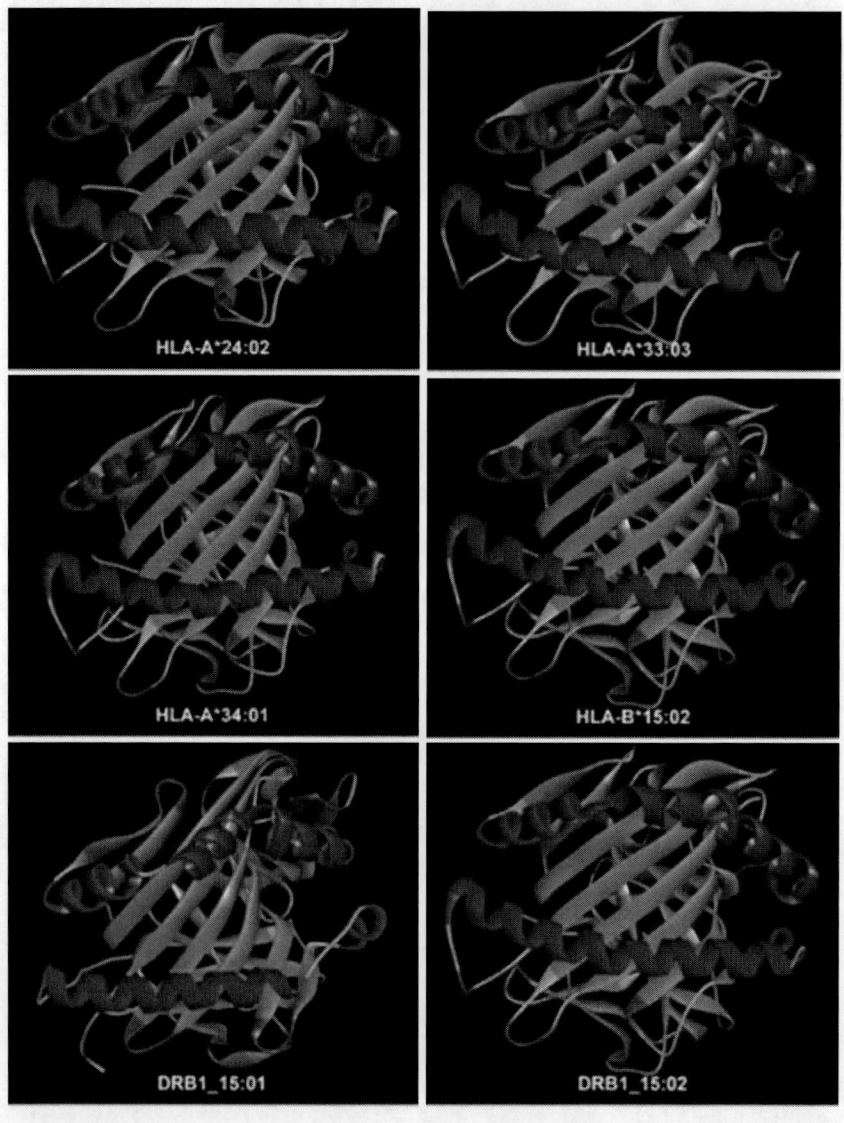

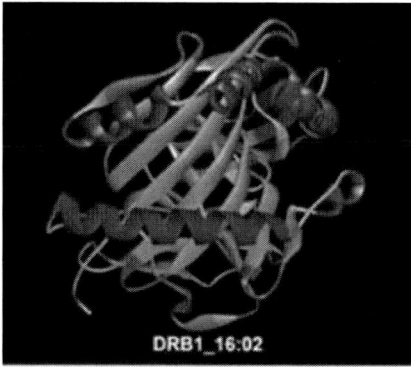

Figure 4. Visualization of MHC molecules from CD4+ and CD8+ T-cells. There are 4 MHC molecules for CD8+ T-cells and 3 MHC molecules for CD4+ T-cells.

Molecular Docking

In order to induce an immune response, proper association between the antigen and immune receptors is essential. HPEPDOCK was used to do the molecular docking for all epitopes and their respective binding partners (Figure 5-6). The binding scores of HTL1-DRB1_15:01 is -235.838 kcal/mol (Figure 5A-B), HTL2-DRB1_15:01 is -243.303 kcal/mol (Figure 5C-D), HTL3-DRB1_15:01 is -238.452 kcal/mol (Figure 5E-F), and HTL4-DRB1_15:01 is -235.902 kcal/mol (Figure 5G-H). The molecular docking analysis for CD4+ epitopes showed effective binding interactions. The binding scores of CTL1-HLA-A*33:03 is -204.707 kcal/mol (Figure 6A-B), CTL2-HLA-A*24:04 is -256.774 kcal/mol (Figure 6C-D), and CTL3-HLA-B*15:02 is -236.909 kcal/mol (Figure 6E-F).

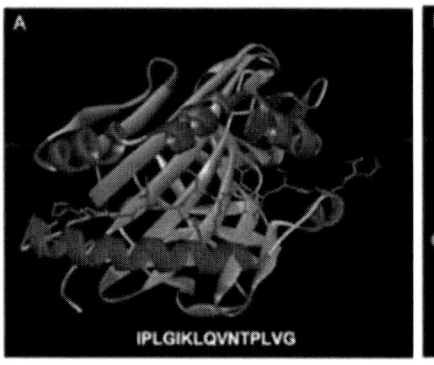
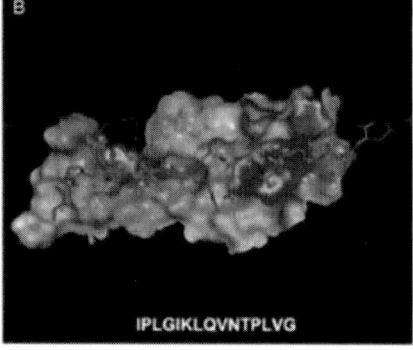

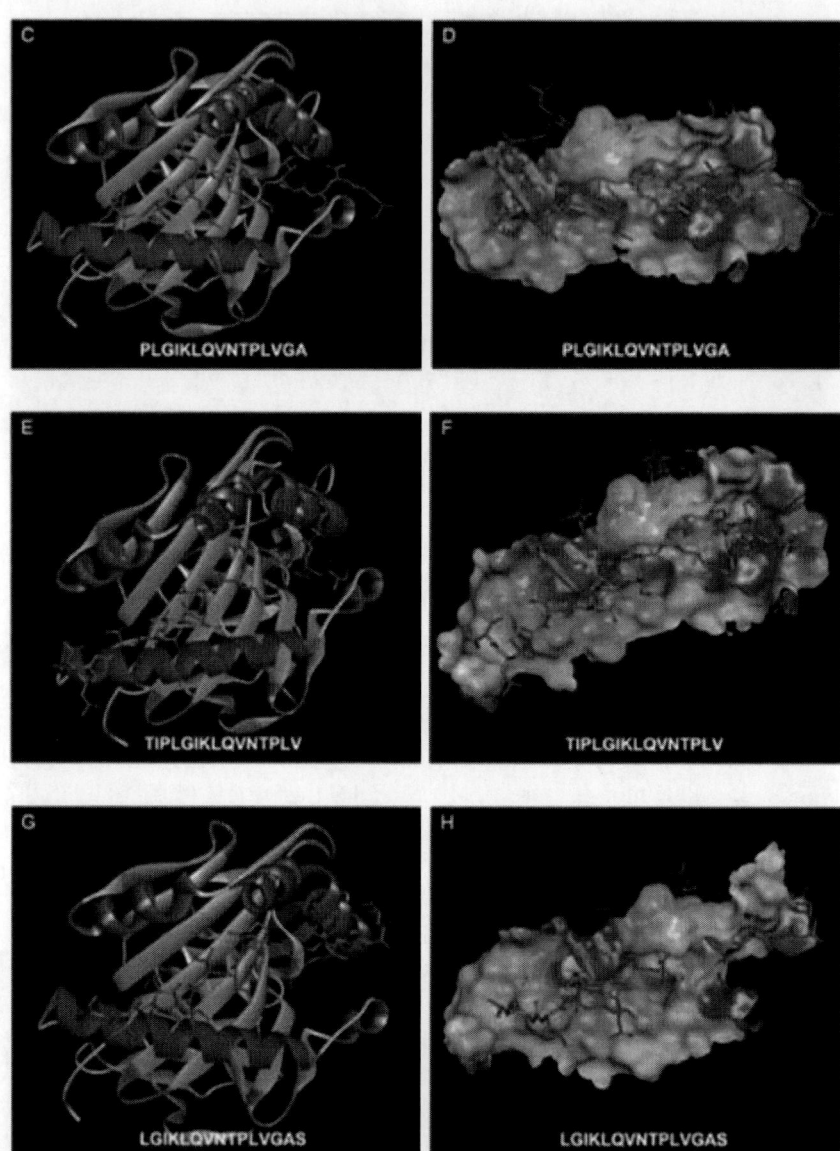

Figure 5. Molecular docking representation of each of the CD8+ epitopes to their respective HLA binding partners. (A) Docking between IPLGIKLQVNTPLVG with DRB1_15:01, (B) Ligand interactions of A, (C) Docking between PLGIKLQVNTPLVGA with DRB1_15:01, (D) Ligand interactions of C, (E) Docking between TIPLGIKLQVNTPLV with DRB1_15:01, (F) Ligand interactions of E, (G) Docking between LGIKLQVNTPLVGAS with DRB1_15:01, (H) Ligand interactions of G.

In Silico Design of a Novel Multi-Epitope Peptide Cancer Vaccine ... 21

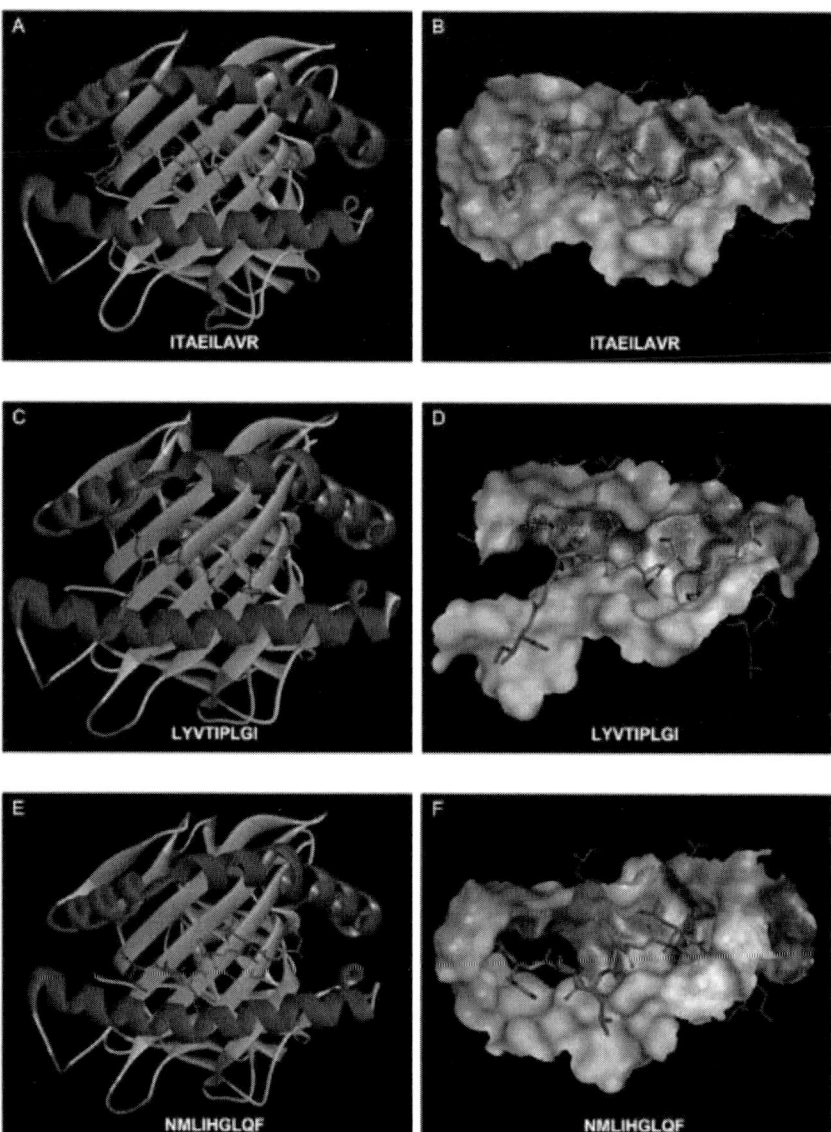

Figure 6. Molecular docking representation of each of the CD4+ epitopes to their respective HLA binding partners. (A) Docking between ITAEILAVR with HLA-A*33:03, (B) Ligand interactions of A, (C) Docking between LYVTIPLGI with HLA-A*24:02, (D) Ligand interactions of C, (E) Docking between NMLIHGLQF with HLA-B*15:02, (F) Ligand interactions of E.

Discussion

NSCLC reportedly requires a particular antigen-targeting approach to increase the efficacy of its treatment due to its pathophysiology, which involves numerous tumour progression mechanisms [12]. The LunX of bactericidal or permeability-increasing protein fold-containing family A member 1 (BPIFA1) is a specific protein found to be overexpressed in NSCLC [20]. Its overexpression is associated with lung cancer migration and proliferation. A previous *in vivo* study revealed that administering anti-LunX slows the growth and metastasis of the NSCLC [21]. Therefore, this study further explored the potential role of LunX as a target antigen for the NSCLC vaccine.

A cancer vaccine needs to be able to induce strong CD4+ and CD8+ T-cell responses [22]. Owing to this fact, this study identified and included both CD4+ and CD8+ epitopes to ensure the vaccine can induce both humoral and cytotoxic immune responses [23]. The CD8+ T-cells will kill the malignant cells directly once they recognize the epitopes presented by the MHC Class I [24]. Meanwhile, the CD4+ T-cells elicit an anti-tumour response by helping the CD8+ T-cells and antibody response [25]. In addition, CD4+ T-cells are also reported to participate in tumour cell killing by secreting effector cytokines, including interferon-γ (IFNγ) and tumour necrosis factor-α (TNFα) [26]. In this study, the epitopes were predicted using NetCTLpan, NetMHCpan, and IEDB antibody binding prediction, which resulted in a total of three final candidates of CD8+ epitopes, four final candidates of CD4+ epitopes, and one final candidate of B-cell epitope to be included in the vaccine construct. All of the epitopes in the vaccine construct are promiscuous, meaning they can bind to multiple HLA and have a positive antigenicity score and IFN score. Moreover, the epitopes included in the vaccine construct have a significant population coverage with a combined (CD4+ and CD8+) score of 95.47%. The estimated population coverage may be more extensive since some of the HLA identified are currently unavailable in the IEDB population tools.

The multi-epitope vaccine was then further linked with an adjuvant, commonly used in vaccines, especially peptide vaccines, to enhance the multi-epitope vaccine activity. Linking the vaccine with the adjuvant induces a proper response generated by dendritic cells [27]. Aside from that, adjuvant was used to enhance the construct's initial physicochemical properties. This study used GM-CSF as the adjuvant, which has been proven to provide sufficient effects towards the multi-epitope tumour vaccine efficacy. GM-CSF was shown to promote potent anti-viral and anti-tumour activities, which support the function of the peptide-based cancer vaccine. The adjuvant's properties resulted from the adjuvant's ability to promote the link between the dendritic cells and T-cells. GM-CSF also activates T-cells through the anti-tumour activity provided by GM-CSF [27-28].

Linkers were then incorporated as they offer various advantages towards the vaccine construct, such as bioactivity enhancement, pharmacokinetic properties suitability induction, and expression yield elevation [29]. Several linkers, including GPGPG, EAAAK, and AAY, were included in the vaccine construct to link the adjuvant, B-cell epitopes, helper T-cell epitopes, and cytotoxic T-cell epitopes while enhancing the epitope presentation to the immune response. The GPGPG linker was used to link all the helper T-cell and B-cell epitopes in the vaccine construct. This linker is considered a flexible linker due to the high content of small and polar glycine amino acid, which provides the flexibility of the conformation for the epitope interaction with the helper T- and B-cells while also distancing the epitopes passively to prevent the neoepitopes formation [29-30]. This specific linker was used since it can stimulate the immune system response, especially helper T-cells and B-cells, towards the epitopes and conserve the conformation-dependent immunogenicity. It mentions that GPGPG is shown to present the epitopes effectively *in vivo* [27, 31]. Another incorporated linker was EAAAK, which linked the GM-CSF adjuvant and the whole multi-epitope vaccine construct by linking with the B-cell epitopes. Due to its rigid properties, EAAAK involves the control of the distance and the interference reduction resulting from the domains of the molecules, which leads to the preservation of the adjuvant bioactivity and stability [27, 29, 31].

Meanwhile, the cytotoxic T-cell epitopes were linked with AAY linkers. After the cleavage process, the AAY linker provides a C-terminal for the proper binding of the TAP transporter of the CD8+ T-cells, which results in improved antigen presentation and optimal antigenicity to the immune cells [27, 32]. Like GPGPG, the AAY linker has been shown to induce effective antigen presentation *in vivo* [31].

The vaccine construct is 281 amino acids long, with a molecular weight of 29858.89 Da and a theoretical pI of 6.89. The results of the physicochemical properties have shown the multi-epitope vaccine to be antigenic, non-allergenic, and stable, which is suitable for further developing the multi-epitope cancer vaccine. Moreover, the GRAVY score of the vaccine construct also indicates that the vaccine is hydrophobic. Thus, it can induce potent T- and B-cell responses [33]. The model of the vaccine construct was then predicted using I-TASSER; model 5 and model 1, with c-scores of -2.52 and

-3.96, respectively, were selected. The c-score indicates confidence level, whereas a higher c-score represents a model with high confidence. The Ramachandran plot found that model 5 is more structurally favourable than model 1, with a favoured value of 73.88%.

Moreover, molecular docking is essential in establishing the vaccine in this study. Molecular docking predicts interactions between protein molecules [34], such as vaccines and HLA molecules. Through molecular docking using HPEPDOCK, it was found that all CD8+ and CD4+ T-cell epitopes exhibit effective binding interactions with their respective HLA molecules.

Conclusion

Lung cancer is the leading cause of cancer-related mortality around the world. The most common type of lung cancer is non-small cell lung cancer (NSCLC). Cancer immunotherapies, specifically vaccines, have been gaining interest among the available therapies due to their specificity. Moreover, multi-epitope peptide cancer vaccines are proven to induce more robust immune responses and cover a larger population. Through immunoinformatics approaches, this work successfully identified and constructed a potential NSCLC cancer vaccine using BPIFA1 antigen that targets specific HLA alleles of the Indonesian population. The vaccine construct can cover many Indonesian populations, has good antigenic and physicochemical properties, and is considered non-allergenic.

Acknowledgment

The authors thank the Department of Research and Community Service (LPPM) of the Indonesia International Institute for Life Sciences for their heartfelt support. Moreover, thanks also go to the Community Language Center of Indonesia International Institute for Life Sciences for their excellent proofreading of our manuscript. The authors declare that there is no competing interest.

References

[1] Molina J. R., Yang P., Cassivi S. D., Schild S. E., Adjei A. A. (2008). Non-small cell lung cancer: Epidemiology, risk factors, treatment, and survivorship. *Mayo Clinic Proceedings*, 83(5):584–94.

[2] Huisman C., Smit E. F., Giaccone G., Postmus P. E. 2000. Second-line chemotherapy in relapsing or refractory non-small-cell lung cancer: A Review. *Journal of Clinical Oncology*, 18(21):3722–30.

[3] Sung H., Ferlay J., Siegel R. L., Laversanne M., Soerjomataram I., Jemal A., Bray F. 2021. Global cancer statistics 2020: Globocan estimates of incidence and mortality worldwide for 36 cancers in 185 countries. *CA: A Cancer Journal for Clinicians*, 71(3):209–49.

[4] Cancer Indonesia 2020 country profile [Internet]. World Health Organization. *World Health Organization*. Available from: https://www.who.int/publications/m/item/cancer-idn-2020.

[5] Hari Kanker Sedunia 2019 [Internet]. *Kementerian Kesehatan Republik Indonesia*. Available from: https://www.kemkes.go.id/article/view/19020100003/hari-kanker-sedunia-2019.html.

[6] Provencio M., Isla D., Sánchez A., Cantos B. 2011. Inoperable stage III non-small cell lung cancer: Current treatment and role of vinorelbine. *J Thorac Dis*, 3(3):197–204.

[7] Anagnostou V. K., Brahmer J. R. 2015. Cancer immunotherapy: A future paradigm shift in treating non–small cell lung cancer. *Clinical Cancer Research*, 21(5):976–84.

[8] Zappa C., Mousa S. A. 2016. Non-small cell lung cancer: Current treatment and future advances. *Translational Lung Cancer Research*, 5(3):288–300.

[9] Schneble E., Clifton G. T., Hale D. F., Peoples G. E. (2016). Peptide-based cancer vaccine strategies and clinical results. *Vaccine Design*, pp. 797–817.

[10] Zhang L. (2017). Multi-epitope vaccines: A promising strategy against tumors and viral infections. *Cellular & Molecular Immunology*, 15(2):182–4.

[11] Sanches R. C., Tiwari S., Ferreira L. C., Oliveira F. M., Lopes M. D., Passos M. J., Maia E. H. D., Taranto A. G., Kato R., Azevedo V. A. C., Lopes D. O. (2021). Immunoinformatics design of multi-epitope peptide-based vaccine against schistosoma mansoni using transmembrane proteins as a target. *Frontiers in Immunology*, 12.

[12] Herrera L. R. (2021). Reverse vaccinology approach in constructing a multi-epitope vaccine against cancer-testis antigens expressed in non-small cell lung cancer. *Asian Pacific Journal of Cancer Prevention*, 22(5):1495–506.

[13] Herrera L. R. (2020). Immuno Informatics Approach in designing a novel vaccine using epitopes from all the structural proteins of SARS-COV-2. *Biomedical and Pharmacology Journal*, 13(4):1845–62.

[14] Lathwal A., Kumar R., Raghava G. P. S. (2021). In-silico identification of subunit vaccine candidates against lung cancer-associated oncogenic viruses. *Computers in Biology and Medicine*, 130:104215.

[15] Krishna S., Anderson K. S. (2016). T-cell epitope discovery for therapeutic cancer vaccines. *Vaccine Design*, pp. 779–96.
[16] Nezafat N., Ghasemi Y., Javadi G., Khoshnoud M. J., Omidinia E. 2014. A novel multi-epitope peptide Vaccine against cancer: An in silico approach. *Journal of Theoretical Biology*, 349:121–34.
[17] Yao B., Zhang L., Liang S., Zhang C. (2012). SVMTriP: A method to predict antigenic epitopes using a support vector machine to integrate tri-peptide similarity and propensity. *PLoS ONE*, 7(9).
[18] Dimitrov I., Bangov I., Flower D. R., Doytchinova I. (2014). AllerTOP V.2—a server for in silico prediction of allergens. *Journal of Molecular Modeling*, 20(6).
[19] Gasteiger E., Hoogland C., Gattiker A., Duvaud S., Wilkins M. R., Appel R. D., Hochstrasser D. F. 2005. Protein identification and analysis tools on the ExPASY server. *The Proteomics Protocols Handbook.*, 571–607.
[20] Wang H., Jiang D., Li W., Wang S. 2017. Increased expression of BPI fold-containing family member 1 is associated with metastasis and poor prognosis in human colorectal carcinoma. *Oncol Lett.*, 14(4):4231–6.
[21] Zheng X., Cheng M., Fu B., Fan X., Wang Q., Yu X., Sun R., Tian Z., Wei H. (2015). Targeting LUNX inhibits non–small cell lung cancer growth and metastasis. *Cancer Research*, 75(6):1080–90.
[22] Oliveres H., Caglevic C., Passiglia F., Taverna S,. Smits E., Rolfo C. 2018. Vaccine and immune cell therapy in non-small cell lung cancer. *Journal of Thoracic Disease*, 10(S13).
[23] Setiawan T., Rizarullah R. 2021. Predicting multi-epitope peptide cancer vaccine from novel Taa Topo48. *Journal of Science and Applicative Technology*, 5(1):171.
[24] Durgeau A., Virk Y., Corgnac S., Mami-Chouaib F. 2018. Recent advances in targeting CD8 T-cell immunity for more effective cancer immunotherapy. *Frontiers in Immunology*, 9.
[25] Tay R. E., Richardson E. K., Toh H. C. (2020). Revisiting the role of CD4+ T cells in cancer immunotherapy—new insights into old paradigms. *Cancer Gene Therapy*, 28(1-2): pp. 5–17.
[26] Melssen M., Slingluff C. L. 2017. Vaccines targeting helper T cells for cancer immunotherapy. *Current Opinion in Immunology*, 47:85–92.
[27] Parvizpour S., Razmara J., Pourseif M. M., Omidi Y. 2018. In silico design of a triple-negative breast cancer vaccine targeting cancer testis antigens. *BioImpacts*, 9(1):45–56.
[28] Zhao W, Zhao G, Wang B. (2017). Revisiting GM-CSF as an adjuvant for therapeutic vaccines. *Cellular & Molecular Immunology*, 15(2):187–9.
[29] Bahrami A. A., Payandeh Z., Khalili S., Zakeri A., Bandehpour M. 2019. Immunoinformatics: In Silico Approaches and computational design of a multi-epitope, immunogenic protein. *International Reviews of Immunology*, 38(6):307–22.
[30] Jafari E., Mahmoodi S. 2021. Design, expression, and purification of a multi-epitope vaccine against helicobacter pylori based on Melittin as an adjuvant. *Microbial Pathogenesis*;157:104970.

[31] Herrera L. R. (2020). In silico approach in designing a novel multi-epitope vaccine candidate against non-small cell lung cancer with overexpressed G protein-coupled receptor 56. *Asian Pacific Journal of Cancer Prevention,* 21(8):2297–306.

[32] Majid M., Andleeb S. 2019. Designing a multi-epitopic vaccine against the enterotoxigenic bacteroides fragilis based on immunoinformatics approach. *Scientific Reports*, 9(1).

[33] Bachmann M. F., Jennings G. T. (2010). Vaccine delivery: A matter of size, geometry, kinetics and molecular patterns. *Nature Reviews Immunology*, 10(11):787–96.

[34] Morris G. M., Lim-Wilby M. (2008). Molecular docking. *Methods in Molecular Biology*, pp. 365–

Chapter 3

The Molecular Docking Approach toward Targeting Transcription Factors in Prostate Cancer

Aileen Gunawan
Joan Nadia
and Arli Aditya Parikesit[*]

Department of Biomedicine, School of Life Sciences, Indonesia International Institute for Life Sciences, Jakarta, Indonesia

Abstract

Cancer is a deadly disease that has accounted for hundreds of thousands of deaths each year around the globe. Prostate cancer is a type of cancer with a high prevalence among men in their sixties. One of the possible causes of this cancer is the mutations in the critical transcriptional factors (TFs) associated with the androgen receptors (ARs), such as FOXA1 and GATA2, which some studies have found to increase the risk of prostate cancer. TFs are one of the most direct and potential targets for treating cancer. However, TFs are very small and have no stable binding sites, which makes it hard to target using small compounds.

Furthermore, limited studies have been conducted to determine the target sites of TFs to treat prostate cancer. This chapter aimed to recount a study approaching natural compound screening against TFs using the conventional molecular docking method. From the molecular docking results and KNApSAcK database, it was found that the natural compound (MolPort-001-742-110_ZINC000059779788) with a binding energy of around -9.6 kcal/mol was present in several herbs containing 2,3-

---

[*] Corresponding Author's Email: arli.parikesit@i3l.ac.id.

In: A Closer Look at Cancer Biomarkers
Editor: Arli Aditya Parikesit
ISBN: 979-8-89113-497-3
© 2024 Nova Science Publishers, Inc.

Dihydroamentoflavone. However, there are still limited studies of the anticancer ability of the herbs. Hence, advanced *in-silico* studies and further wet lab activities, including *in-vitro* and *in-vivo* studies, are required to evaluate and expand these findings.

Keywords: prostate cancer, transcription factors, molecular docking, drug target, natural compound

Introduction

In 2012, nearly 14 million new cancer cases were diagnosed worldwide, resulting in approximately 8.2 million deaths. Prostate cancer is the most common malignant neoplasm affecting men, especially in their sixth decade of life (Takayama et al., 2021; Simoes et al., 2018). The prostate gland is a male sexual gland in front of the rectum and between the bladder and the penis (Daniyal et al., 2014). The development of prostate cancer involves the corruption of the normal prostate transcriptional network due to deregulated expression or mutation of crucial transcription factors (Bushweller, 2019). Currently, a few ways to treat cancer include surgery, radical prostatectomy, medication, and cytotoxic chemotherapy (Daniyal et al., 2014; Teo et al., 2019). However, these treatments often cause side effects, such as impotence, urinary disturbance, complications, or even death. Consequently, a new alternative way needs to be found to treat cancer with the least prevalence of inducing severe side effects. Targeting the transcription factor (TF) is known to be a promising way to treat cancer, yet very little active research has been conducted regarding this treatment (Bushweller, 2019).

In recent years, natural compounds have been studied to possess anticancer effects, which are safer than synthetic compounds (Gullett et al., 2010). Using natural compounds is known to suppress the growth and inhibit the metastasis of the cancer cells, including prostate cancer. Moreover, these compounds can target the androgen receptors associated with specific cancer (Fontana et al., 2020). In addition, most natural compounds may induce reactive oxygen species (ROS) that increase the vulnerability of the cancer cells (Tang et al., 2014). Androgens and the androgen receptor (AR) have been shown to play a significant role in prostate cancer progression. Some AR collaborative TFs, such as GATA binding protein 2 (GATA2) and forkhead box A1 (FOXA1), stimulate AR activity in the castration-resistant state, according to functional molecular studies (Yuan et al., 2019). However, there have been limited studies regarding the use of natural compounds for prostate cancer treatment. Hence, this chapter is done to determine the possible lead-like drug from natural compounds that target the TFs to treat prostate cancer via *an in silico* approach using molecular docking analysis.

Methods

Data Retrieval

Data was retrieved from NCBI and PDB databases. The FASTA sequences of FOXA1 and GATA2 derived from *Homo sapiens* were retrieved from the NCBI database (https://www.ncbi.nlm.nih.gov/). The PDB files needed for molecular docking analysis (Schneidman-Duhovny et al., 2005) were downloaded through AlphaFold (https://alphafold.ebi.ac.uk/) and PDB (https://www.rcsb.org/) for FOXA1 and GATA2, respectively.

Binding Domain Domain Binding Selection

The possible binding domain of the transcription factor protein was then determined using the Interpro website (https://www.ebi.ac.uk/interpro/). Following each hit of a protein sequence, several parameters were obtained, including the 'domain' parameter.

Molecular Docking-Screening

The screening was performed through molecular docking using MTIOpenScreen (https://bioserv.rpbs.univ-paris-diderot.fr/services/MTiOpenScreen/). The PDB of each transcription factor domain was inputted into the protein receptor column in the respective program. The natural product (NP-lib) compound database was chosen in open settings. The program's default settings were then used for running the docking analysis. Through force-field scoring, the obtained scoring function was used to analyze the binding affinity between the drug molecules and transcription factors (Tanchuk et al., 2016). The compound with the highest negative binding score was proposed as the drug model candidate to deal with prostate cancer disease.

Herbal Compound Retrieval

The MolPort ID of the proposed compound was then searched on the MolPort website (https://www.molport.com/) to obtain its molecular formula. Afterwards, the KNApSAcK database (http://www.knapsackfamily.com/KNApSAcK_Family/) was used to find additional information regarding the availability of the compound in nature, such as the name of the metabolites and also the organism in which it can be found.

Results

Through the PDB validation, it was observed that these two sequences were of a complete sequence (Table 1) with a domain binding site, in which these sites would be used for molecular docking (Table 2).

Table 1. The sequences retrieved for FOXA1 and GATA2

No.	Transcription factors	Accession ID	Sample Name	Database
1.	FOXA1	NP_004487.2	hepatocyte nuclear factor 3-alpha [Homo sapiens]	NCBI
2.	GATA2	NP_001139133.1	Endothelial transcription factor GATA-2 isoform 1 [Homo sapiens]	NCBI

Table 2. Domain binding site for FOXA1 and GATA2

No.	Transcription factors	Domain binding site
1.	FOXA1	DNA-binding site
2.	GATA2	DNA-binding site, Zinc-binding site

From Tables 3 and 4, the natural compound with the compound ID of MolPort-001-742-110_ZINC000059779788 was shown to have the highest negative binding energy with a value of -9.7 and -9.3 kcal/mol towards FOXA1 and GATA2, respectively. However, it did not differ significantly from the other compounds against GATA2.

Table 3. Binding energies of natural compounds towards FOXA1

No.	Compound	Binding Energy (kcal/mol)
1	MolPort-001-742-110_ZINC000059779788	-9.7
2.	MolPort-039-338-696_ZINC000299817665	-9.0
3.	MolPort-027-835-585_ZINC000004027386	-8.8
4.	MolPort-027-836-471_ZINC000242547689	-8.8
5.	MolPort-035-705-955_ZINC000003594862	-8.8

Table 4. Binding energies of natural compounds towards GATA2

No.	Compound	Binding Energy (kcal/mol)
1.	MolPort-001-742-110_ZINC000059779788	-9.3
2.	MolPort-001-740-100_ZINC000000603253	-9.3
3.	MolPort-035-705-955_ZINC000003594862	-9.2
4.	MolPort-039-052-621_ZINC000044404209	-9.2
5.	MolPort-003-983-881_ZINC000004517154	-8.8

Table 5. The compound details of MolPort-001-742-110_ZINC000059779788

CAS ID	IUPAC Name	Molecular Formula	Molecular Weight
34340-51-7	(8-[(2S)-5,7-dihydroxy-2-(4-hydroxyphenyl)-4-oxo-2,3-dihydrochromen-8-yl]-5,7-dihydroxy-2-(4-hydroxyphenyl)chromen-4-one	$C_{30}H_{20}O_{10}$	540.48

Table 6. Possible organisms from the KNApSAcK database

No.	CAS ID	Metabolite	Molecular Formula	Molecular Weight	Organisms
1.	34340-51-7	2,3-Dihydroamentoflavone	$C_{30}H_{20}O_{10}$	540.105	*Cycas revoluta*
2.	34340-51-7	2,3-Dihydroamentoflavone	$C_{30}H_{20}O_{10}$	540.105	*Libocedrus bidwillii*
3.	34340-51-7	2,3-Dihydroamentoflavone	$C_{30}H_{20}O_{10}$	540.105	*Libocedrus plumosa*

Through the KNApSAcK database, it was observed that the metabolites of 2,3-Dihydroamentoflavone have the same CAS ID, and yet, there was a minimal difference between the molecular weights. The analysis found three organisms, *Cycas revoluta, Libocedrus bidwillii,* and *Libocedrus plumosa,* where this metabolite could be found. These herbal compounds could be used for further research on their anticancer ability to target the transcription factors in prostate cancer treatment (Table 5 and 6).

Discussion

Molecular docking can be used to analyze the binding site and orientation of the ligand during protein-ligand interactions (Meng et al., 2011). One of its applications is to investigate the potential leads of the drug targeting the binding site of the transcription factors (Pagadala et al., 2017). In this chapter, the sequences of the transcription factors were taken from the NCBI database for domain selection, which was then downloaded as a program database (PDB) file for molecular docking analysis (Schneidman-Duhovny et al., 2005). Through molecular docking analysis, the binding energy was obtained from each sequence towards the natural compound database, in which the one with the highest negative energy was further analyzed to check for possible herbal compounds through KNApSAcK.

Before molecular docking, the domain binding selection of the obtained sequence was conducted to aid in predicting the possible protein intra-domain for the ligand to bind and exert its biological processes (Sigrist et al., 2010). It was found that the FOXA1 possessed a DNA-binding site, and GATA2 possessed a DNA-binding site and zinc-binding site (Table 2). Transcription factors use the DNA-binding to bind to DNA (Si et al., 2015). The binding of a transcription factor to its complementary DNA sequence is considered to be specific (Inukai et al., 2017). Meanwhile, the zinc-binding site is defined as a simple structure comprising an α-helix and a β-sheet that are held together by zinc to form a cluster. This precedent will, in turn, allow each helix to be in contact with the major groove of the DNA, forming a nearly continuous stretch of helices along the groove. These binding motives are site-specific when binding to DNA (Ireland & Martin, 2019). These two binding sites are frequently associated with specialized proteins known as transcription factors, which were the focus of this project to be further analyzed in docking (Figure 1).

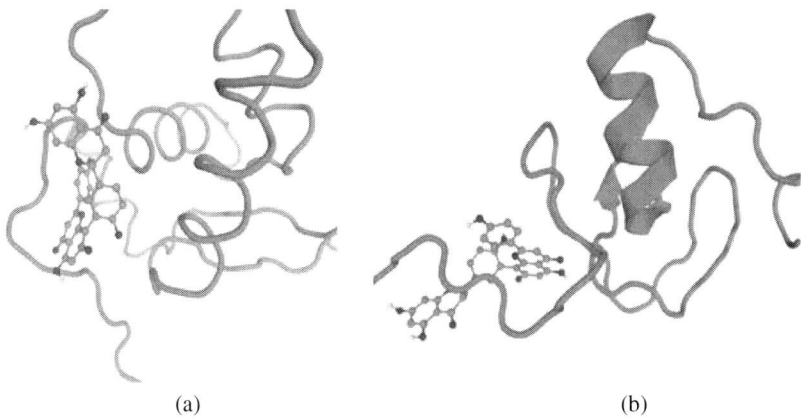

Figure 1. 3D Visualization of a) FOXA1 and b) GATA2 docked with MolPort-001-742-110_ZINC000059779788 by OpenMTI.

Binding energy is one of the parameters that help select a potential drug or ligand candidate (Claveria-Gimeno et al., 2017). Like Gibbs free energy, a negative binding energy value means the reaction occurs spontaneously without energy consumption (Du et al., 2016). From Tables 3 and 4, the natural compound with the compound ID of MolPort-001-742-110_ZINC0000 59779788 was a compound shared in common between the two proteins returning most negative binding energy with a value of -9.7 and -9.3 kcal/mol towards FOXA1 and GATA2, respectively. According to Gurung et al. (2016), an excellent protein-ligand interaction should have a binding energy between -8.0 kcal/mol and -11.71 kcal/mol. In addition, a higher specificity of protein-ligand interaction is achieved when there is a significant negative binding energy within the previously mentioned range (Claveria-Gimeno et al., 2017). In another study using different compounds, it was observed that the highest binding affinity was -9.6 kcal/mol, which was similar to the experimental result from this chapter (Nogueira et al., 2021). Comparing the top five results of the natural compound with the most significant negative binding energy towards both transcription factors was then utilized to screen the potential herbal compounds.

The resulting compound 2,3-Dihydroamentoflavone was considered a candidate inhibitor for the transcriptional factors, in which this metabolite might be found in *Cycas revoluta* and *Librocedrus* genus plants. *Cycas revoluta*, also known as the Sago palm, is a gymnosperm species in the Cycadaceae family used in traditional Medicine. The chemical constituents and crude extracts, especially on the plant leaves, have been shown to have anticancer properties. However, some studies mentioned that these plants might severely threaten human health (Prakash et al., 2020). Aside from the Sago palm, it was also discovered in two members of the Cupressaceae family plants under the *Libocedrus* genus. However, the medicinal uses of both of these compounds were recently discovered when there is still no record of their anticancer ability.

Therefore, further research, especially wet lab experiments, still needs to be conducted to validate these docking results toward inhibiting the cancer progression since the binding energies towards the transcription factors were still in the range for efficient protein-ligand interactions. In addition, the active site of the domain binding site was not analyzed in this experiment due to the limitation of the online website; hence, it is suggested that the predicted active site of the transcription factors would be determined to further validate the interactions through PyMOL or CastP in future experiments.

Conclusion

This chapter attempted to use the molecular docking approach to screen natural compounds for potential inhibitors against the transcription factors FOXA1 and GATA2, especially of relevance in prostate cancer. The compound 2,3-Dihydroamentoflavone was found to dock to both TFs based on the binding energy. The research should be continued with wet lab experiments to confirm the inhibitory activities of the compound.

Acknowledgment

The authors thank the Department of Research and Community Service (LPPM) of the Indonesia International Institute for Life Sciences for their heartfelt support. Moreover, thanks also go to the Community Language Center of Indonesia International Institute for Life Sciences for their excellent proofreading of our manuscript. The authors declare that there is no competing interest.

References

Bushweller, J. H. (2019). Targeting transcription factors in cancer—from undruggable to reality. *Nature Reviews Cancer, 19*(11), 611-624. https://doi.org/10.1038/s41568-019-0196-7.

Claveria-Gimeno, R., Vega, S., Abian, O., Velazquez-Campoy, A. (2017). A look at ligand binding thermodynamics in drug discovery. *Expert Opinion on Drug Discovery, 12*(4), 363-377. https://doi.org/10.1080/17460441.2017.1297418.

Daniyal, M., Siddiqui, Z., Akram, M., Asif, H., Sultana, S., Khan, A. (2014). Epidemiology, Etiology, Diagnosis and Treatment of Prostate Cancer. *Asian Pacific Journal of Cancer Prevention, 15*(22), 9575-9578. https://doi.org/10.7314/apjcp.2014.15.22.9575.

Du, X., Li, Y., Xia, Y. L., Ai, S. M., Liang, J., Sang, P., ... & Liu, S. Q. (2016). Insights into protein–ligand interactions: mechanisms, models, and methods. *International journal of molecular sciences, 17*(2), 144. https://doi.org/10.3390%2Fijms17020144.

Fontana, F., Raimondi, M., Marzagalli, M., Di Domizio, A., Limonta, P. (2020). Natural compounds in prostate cancer prevention and treatment: mechanisms of action and molecular targets. *Cells, 9*(2), 460. https://doi.org/10.3390/cells9020460.

Gullett, N. P., Amin, A. R., Bayraktar, S., Pezzuto, J. M., Shin, D. M., Khuri, F. R., ... & Kucuk, O. (2010, June). Cancer prevention with natural compounds. In *Seminars in oncology* (Vol. 37, No. 3, pp. 258-281). WB Saunders. https://doi.org/10.1053/j.seminoncol.2010.06.014.

Gurung, A. B., Bhattacharjee, A., Ali, M. A. (2016). Exploring the physicochemical profile and the binding patterns of selected novel anticancer Himalayan plant-derived active compounds with macromolecular targets. *Informatics in Medicine Unlocked, pp. 5*, 1–14. https://doi.org/10.1016/j.imu.2016.09.004.

Inukai, S., Kock, K. H., Bulyk, M. L. (2017). Transcription factor–DNA binding: beyond binding site motifs. *Current opinion in genetics & development, 43*, 110-119. https://doi.org/10.1016%2Fj.gde.2017.02.007.

Ireland, S. M., & Martin, A. C. R. (2019). ZincBind-the database of zinc-binding sites. *Database, 2019*, baz006. https://doi.org/10.1093/database/baz006.

Meng, X. Y., Zhang, H. X., Mezei, M., Cui, M. (2011). Molecular docking: a powerful approach for structure-based drug discovery. *Current computer-aided drug design, 7*(2), 146-157. https://doi.org/10.2174%2F157340911795677602.

Nogueira, J. R., Verza, F. A., Nishimura, F., Das, U., Caruso, Í. P., Fachin, A. L., ... & Marins, M. (2021). Molecular Docking Studies of Curcumin Analogues against SARS-CoV-2 Spike Protein. *Journal of the Brazilian Chemical Society, 32*, 1943-1955. https://doi.org/10.21577/0103-5053.20210085.

Pagadala, N. S., Syed, K., Tuszynski, J. (2017). Software for molecular docking: a review. *Biophysical reviews, 9*(2), 91-102. https://doi.org/10.1007/s12551-016-0247-1.

Prakash, V., Kaur, H., Kumari, A.R., Kumar, M., Bala, R., Gupta, S. (2020). Phytochemicals and biological studies on *Cycas revoluta* Thunb.: a review. *Advances in Traditional Medicine, pp. 21*, 389–404. https://doi.org/10.1007/s13596-020-00520-z.

Schneidman-Duhovny, D., Inbar, Y., Nussinov, R., Wolfson, H. J. (2005). PatchDock and SymmDock: servers for rigid and symmetric docking. *Nucleic acids research, 33*(suppl_2), W363-W367. https://doi.org/10.1093/nar/gki481.

Si, J., Zhao, R., Wu, R. (2015). An overview of the prediction of protein DNA-binding sites. *International journal of molecular sciences, 16*(3), 5194–5215. https://doi.org/10.3390/ijms16035194.

Sigrist, C. J., Cerutti, L., de Castro, E., Langendijk-Genevaux, P. S., Bulliard, V., Bairoch, A., Hulo, N. (2010). PROSITE, a protein domain database for functional characterization and annotation. *Nucleic acids research, 38*(Database issue), D161–D166. https://doi.org/10.1093/nar/gkp885.

Simoes, G., Sakuramoto, P., Santos, C., Furlan, N., Augusto, T. (2018). An Overview on Prostate Pathophysiology: New Insights into Prostate Cancer Clinical Diagnosis. *Pathophysiology - Altered Physiological States.* https://doi.org/10.5772/intechopen.74269.

Takayama, K. I., Kosaka, T., Suzuki, T., Hongo, H., Oya, M., Fujimura, T., ... & Inoue, S. (2021). Subtype-specific collaborative transcription factor networks are promoted by OCT4 in the progression of prostate cancer. *Nature Communications, 12*(1), 1-16. https://doi.org/10.1038/s41467-021-23974-4.

Tanchuk, V. Y., Tanin, V. O., Vovk, A. I., Poda, G. (2016). A new, improved hybrid scoring function for molecular docking and scoring based on AutoDock and AutoDock Vina. *Chemical biology & drug design, 87*(4), 618-625. https://doi.org/10.1111/cbdd.12697.

Tang, Y., Chen, R., Huang, Y., Li, G., Huang, Y., Chen, J., ... & Li, B. (2014). Natural compound alternol induces oxidative stress–dependent apoptotic cell death preferentially in prostate cancer cells. *Molecular cancer therapeutics, 13*(6), 1526-1536. https://doi.org/10.1158/1535-7163.MCT-13-0981.

Teo, M. Y., Rathkopf, D. E., Kantoff, P. (2019). Treatment of advanced prostate cancer. *Annual Review of Medicine, 70,* 479-499. https://doi.org/10.1146/annurev-med-051517-011947.

Yuan, F., Hankey, W., Wu, D., Wang, H., Somarelli, J., Armstrong, A. J., Huang, J., Chen, Z., Wang, Q. (2019). Molecular determinants for enzalutamide-induced transcription in prostate cancer. *Nucleic acids research, 47*(19), 10104–10114. https://doi.org/10.1093/nar/gkz790.

Chapter 4

A Closer Look at Cancer Biomarkers: Their Updated Uses for the Diagnosis and Treatment of Cancer

Carlos A. González Núñez[1,*], MD
Daniel A. García Padilla[2], MD
and Alberto Monroy Chargoy[3], MD

[1]Instituto Nacional de Cancerología, Ciudad de México, México
[2]ONKIMIA, Guadalajara, Jalisco, México
[3]Hospital Regional de Alta Especialidad de Ixtapalauca, Ixtapaluca, Estado de México

Abstract

Cancer has become a public health problem in the last decade, represent the second most common cause of death in the United States. With an estimate of 609,360 deaths from cancer expected in the US in 2022, calculating 1,670 deaths per day. Considering this relevant problem, different strategies have been implemented to change this paradigm. Although a challenge, research for different biomarkers as a screening method to detect neoplasms such as breast, lung, colon, and stomach cancer has been studied. Although several screening strategies are currently available to detect the most common types of cancer, there is still some debate in its impact on mortality, an example could be prostate cancer antigen. This blood test is associated with earlier detection of prostate cancer with debate in its impact on mortality. Accumulation of epigenetic and genetic changes could lead to irregularities in the proteins expressed by the affected cells causing cancer. These changes could be

---

[*] Corresponding Author: drgonzalez.oncologia@gmail.com.

In: A Closer Look at Cancer Biomarkers
Editor: Arli Aditya Parikesit
ISBN: 979-8-89113-497-3
© 2024 Nova Science Publishers, Inc.

detected by biomarkers that could analysis gen variations, as well as alterations in messenger RNA or protein expression. Although this appears like a practice changing diagnosis method, these tests are currently in investigation.

Biomarkers can also guide our treatment in those diagnosed with cancer, helping establish a prognosis, and even deescalating certain treatments. To set an example, Oncotype Dx is a genetic firm that analyses 21 genes to establish if the patient has risk for recurrence. This genetic test has helped reduce the number of patients receiving chemotherapy, due to a lower genetic risk of recurrence. Next Generation Sequencing (NGS) technologies are another example that includes a spectrum of genomic alterations; including mutations, copy number variations, and fusion of multiple genes which will help determine certain therapies (2). This diagnostic test approved for certain types of cancer, lung cancer, prostate cancer, etc. has allowed to provide biomarker directed and targeted therapy. In this chapter we will review have a closer look at the role of biomarkers as an additional form to diagnosis cancer, it´s prognostic value, and the changes in treatment due to the results in different biomarkers.

Keywords: cancer, biomarker, diagnosis, prevention, precision medicine, targeted therapy, screening

Introduction

Over the past decade, cancer has emerged as a pressing public health concern, ranking as the second leading cause of death in the United States. The grim statistics project an estimated 609,360 cancer-related deaths in the US for 2022, translating to an alarming average of 1,670 lives lost daily [1]. Recognizing the gravity of this issue, many strategies have been set in motion to reshape this troubling narrative. Among these endeavours, investigating biomarkers as a screening tool for detecting neoplasms like breast, lung, colon, and stomach cancer has garnered significant attention [2].

While several screening methods are currently available for the most prevalent cancer types, a lingering debate surrounds their impact on mortality, exemplified by the case of prostate cancer antigen testing. This blood test is linked to the earlier detection of prostate cancer, yet its ultimate effect on mortality remains a subject of contention [3]. The underlying cause of cancer often lies in the accumulation of epigenetic and genetic alterations, leading to disruptions in the proteins expressed by affected cells. Biomarkers capable of scrutinizing genetic variations and alterations in messenger RNA or protein expression hold promise in identifying these changes [4]. However, it is important to note that while these diagnostic approaches appear game-changers, they are still in the investigative phase.

Biomarkers also play a pivotal role in guiding the treatment of individuals diagnosed with cancer, aiding in prognosis determination, and even facilitating the reduction of certain treatment interventions. For instance, consider Oncotype Dx, a genetic analysis firm that assesses 21 specific genes to ascertain a patient's risk of cancer recurrence. This genetic test has effectively contributed to a decrease in the number of patients undergoing chemotherapy, especially for those with a lower genetic risk of recurrence [5].

Another noteworthy advancement is the application of Next Generation Sequencing (NGS) technologies, encompassing a spectrum of genomic alterations, including mutations, copy number variations, and fusion of multiple genes. These technologies prove instrumental in tailoring specific therapies for patients [2]. This diagnostic test, approved for select cancer types like lung and prostate cancer, has paved the way for biomarker-directed and targeted therapy [6].

In the upcoming chapter, we will delve more deeply into biomarkers as an additional tool for cancer diagnosis, their prognostic significance, and the consequential treatment modifications based on diverse biomarker findings.

Biomarkers as a Screening Tool

Cancer screening recommendations usually start by age 40 to detect cancer at an early and curable stage [7, 8]. Although current screening recommendations have helped curve the prognosis in certain types of cancer, screening is not available for most types of cancer. In recent years, blood-based cancer assays have evolved, detecting protein, microRNA, circulating tumour DNA, and methylated DNA biomarkers, which are used in more advanced cancers and have helped shift therapeutic decisions [7].

Circulating miRNA has emerged as a promising diagnostic tool for screening. These miRNAs play a pivotal role in regulating various cellular processes, including growth, apoptosis, proliferation, and differentiation. Any disruption in their normal function can potentially lead to cancer development. Dysregulation of miRNAs in cancer can be attributed to biogenesis, expression, or function alterations. These alterations may result in the overexpression or underexpression of specific miRNAs, contributing to cancer's onset and progression. Consequently, extensive research has been conducted to investigate the potential of miRNAs as biomarkers for cancer detection and monitoring [9].

Numerous studies have demonstrated the utility of miRNAs as biomarkers for cancer screening. For instance, a study published in "Cancer Epidemiology, Biomarkers & Prevention" identified four miRNAs that could accurately distinguish between individuals with lung cancer and healthy controls [10]. Similarly, another study published in the journal "Oncotarget" pinpointed a panel of five miRNAs as a potential biomarker for prostate cancer [11].

One advantage of using miRNAs as biomarkers for cancer is their stability in bodily fluids. miRNAs can be detected in blood, urine, and other bodily fluids, making them a non-invasive and easily accessible biomarker for cancer screening.

Despite their potential as biomarkers for cancer screening, challenges still need to be addressed before miRNAs can be used in clinical practice. These challenges include the lack of standardized protocols for miRNA detection and quantification, as well as the need for large-scale validation studies [12].

In conclusion, miRNAs are promising biomarkers for cancer screening and monitoring. Further research is needed to validate their utility in clinical practice and to address the challenges associated with their detection and quantification.

Another method that is now FDA-approved is epigenetics to detect certain types of cancer, such as colorectal cancer. Epigenetics, the study of inheritable changes in gene expression without alterations to the DNA sequence itself, has emerged as a promising approach for cancer screening. By examining reversible modifications to DNA and histones, epigenetic alterations offer valuable insights into early cancer detection and risk assessment. This essay delves into the potential of epigenetics as a cancer screening method, emphasizing its advantages and referencing pertinent studies [12].

Epigenetic changes can manifest at various stages of carcinogenesis, providing valuable biomarkers for cancer screening. One notable example is the observation of aberrant DNA methylation patterns in several cancer types, including colorectal, breast, and lung cancer. Screening assays based on DNA methylation, such as methylation-specific PCR and bisulfite sequencing, have demonstrated promising results in detecting cancer-specific methylation patterns.

Histone modifications also play a crucial role in cancer development and progression. Altered patterns of histone acetylation, methylation, and phosphorylation have been associated with various types of cancer. Chromatin immunoprecipitation assays coupled with next-generation sequencing can identify and characterize these histone modifications, providing valuable information for cancer screening [11].

Epigenetic screening offers several advantages. First, it enables early cancer detection by identifying epigenetic alterations in the early stages of tumorigenesis, even before clinical symptoms manifest. Early detection improves treatment outcomes and patient survival rates.

Second, epigenetic screening can be non-invasive, as epigenetic modifications can be detected in body fluids such as blood, urine, saliva, and faeces. Non-invasive sampling reduces patient discomfort, increases participation rates, and allows population-wide screening efforts.

Lastly, epigenetic alterations exhibit tissue-specific patterns, making them valuable for organ-specific cancer screening. Analyzing tissue-specific epigenetic markers enables the identification of cancerous changes in specific organs, enhancing the accuracy and efficiency of screening protocols [12].

While the potential of epigenetic cancer screening is promising, there are challenges to overcome. Standardizing methodologies, robust biomarkers identification, and screening assay validation are crucial for clinical implementation. Large-scale prospective studies and collaboration between researchers, clinicians, and industry partners are necessary to establish the clinical utility, cost-effectiveness, and integration of epigenetic screening into routine cancer management.

In conclusion, epigenetics offers a promising method for cancer screening by providing valuable insights into early detection and risk assessment. Identifying epigenetic alterations through DNA methylation and histone modifications allows for the development of sensitive and specific screening assays. However, further research and validation are needed to establish the clinical utility of epigenetic screening in routine cancer management [13].

Biomarkers in Lung Cancer

Lung cancer is among the most common and deadly cancers worldwide [13]. The early detection and treatment of lung cancer is essential for improving patient outcomes. Biomarkers have emerged as important tools in the diagnosis and therapeutic management of lung cancer.

Biomarkers are measurable characteristics that indicate the presence or severity of a disease. In lung cancer, biomarkers can be used for diagnosis, prognosis, and prediction of response to therapy. The most commonly used biomarkers in lung cancer include genetic mutations, protein expression, and circulating tumour cells.

One of the most renowned biomarkers in the context of lung cancer is the epidermal growth factor receptor (EGFR) mutation. These EGFR mutations are found in approximately 10-15% of non-small cell lung cancers (NSCLCs). What makes EGFR mutations significant is their strong responsiveness to EGFR tyrosine kinase inhibitors (TKIs), such as gefitinib and erlotinib. These TKIs are targeted therapies designed to inhibit EGFR activity effectively [14].

However, within the group of individuals with EGFR mutations, those who also carry a T790M mutation can develop resistance to 1st and 2nd-generation EGFR TKI therapies, either through acquired resistance or de novo resistance [15]. Identifying the T790M mutation becomes crucial as it can guide treatment choices in the first-line or second-line therapeutic settings.

The T790M mutation can be detected through various methods, including tissue biopsy, liquid biopsy, and the analysis of circulating tumour DNA (ctDNA). Of note, liquid biopsy and ctDNA analysis stand out for their less invasive nature and the ability to perform more frequently than traditional tissue biopsies [16]. These less intrusive methods offer a practical advantage in the ongoing monitoring and management of EGFR mutations in lung cancer patients.

Another biomarker is ALK, or anaplastic lymphoma kinase, which plays a critical role in diagnosing and treating non-small cell lung cancer (NSCLC). ALK is a receptor tyrosine kinase involved in various cellular processes, including cell growth and proliferation. In NSCLC, ALK gene rearrangements result in the expression of fusion proteins that drive cancer growth and progression.

ALK gene rearrangements are present in approximately 3-5% of NSCLC cases and are more commonly found in younger patients and non-smokers [17].

Identifying ALK rearrangements as a biomarker in non-small cell lung cancer (NSCLC) has paved the way for developing targeted therapies. These therapies, known as ALK inhibitors, specifically target the fusion protein responsible for driving cancer growth.

The first ALK inhibitor approved for treating ALK-positive NSCLC was crizotinib. Subsequent generations of ALK inhibitors have since been developed, including ceritinib, alectinib, and brigatinib. These inhibitors have demonstrated impressive response rates and extended progression-free survival in patients diagnosed with ALK-positive NSCLC [18, 19].

It is advisable to conduct ALK testing in all patients with advanced NSCLC, especially those with a history of never smoking or a younger age at diagnosis [20]. Various methods are available for detecting ALK rearrangements, including fluorescence in situ hybridization (FISH), immunohistochemistry (IHC), and next-generation sequencing (NGS). FISH is considered the gold standard for ALK testing, but IHC and NGS have emerged as viable alternatives, offering similar sensitivity and specificity [21]. These options provide flexibility in selecting the most appropriate method for ALK testing based on individual patient characteristics and laboratory capabilities.

Another biomarker commonly used in lung cancer is programmed death-ligand 1 (PD-L1). PD-L1 is an immune checkpoint protein that is overexpressed in some types of cancer, including lung cancer. The expression of PD-L1 in tumour cells is associated with an increased response to immune checkpoint inhibitors, such as pembrolizumab and nivolumab [22].

Circulating tumour cells (CTCs) represent a crucial biomarker in lung cancer. These tumour cells detached from the primary tumour and entered the bloodstream. The detection of CTCs in blood samples has been linked to disease progression and a less favourable prognosis in lung cancer patients [23].

In summary, biomarkers have become indispensable tools in the diagnosis and therapeutic management of lung cancer, significantly altering the prognosis. Their utilization has led to enhanced patient outcomes and the development of personalized treatment strategies. Further research is essential to identify novel biomarkers and validate their clinical utility in lung cancer.

The realm of biomarkers continues to evolve and offers promising opportunities in lung cancer, significantly impacting patient survival through tailored therapeutic options. Genomic platforms like next-generation sequencing have received category-one recommendations in international guidelines, such as the updated 2023 NCCN Non-Small Cell Lung Cancer guidelines. These platforms are utilized to detect a range of biomarkers, including EGFR, ALK, KRAS, ROS1, BRAF, NTRK1/2/3, METex14 skipping, RET, ERBB2 (HER2), and the expression of PD-L1, thus guiding directed therapeutic decisions for patients. The detection of PD-L1 and EGFR is also recommended in patients with locally advanced disease, as it influences various therapeutic options, including adjuvant Atezolizumab and Osimertinib, respectively [24].

Biomarkers in Genitourinary Neoplasms

Kidney Cancer

Despite the rising incidence of kidney cancer in recent years and significant advancements in treating advanced kidney cancer (including combinations of immunotherapy and targeted therapy), a critical challenge persists without a reliable biomarker to predict treatment response. Consequently, ongoing research in kidney cancer remains dedicated to identifying such biomarkers [25].

For a considerable duration, the IMDC classification has served as the primary means to assess the prognosis of kidney cancer patients and even determine suitable treatment approaches. In the tyrosine kinase inhibitors (TKIs) era, this classification has formed the basis for most modern clinical trials focused on first-line treatment [26]. However, the quest for biomarkers that can provide more precise prognostic insights for patients with this disease is ongoing.

One notable observation is that in certain clinical trials utilizing immunotherapy, tumours exhibiting PD-L1 positivity have shown improved survival rates. Regrettably, only 26% of tumors express this biomarker [27].

The von Hippel-Lindau (VHL) tumour suppressor gene, specifically the VHL170 variant, is frequently altered in kidney cancer cases, with bi-allelic inactivation occurring in roughly 60 to 90% of instances. This alteration significantly contributes to the development of tumours, angiogenesis, and changes in the tumour microenvironment [28]. Although the VHL/HIF/VEGF pathway holds promise as a potential target for therapies, currently, anti-angiogenic treatments appear to be the primary option with limited anti-tumor activity [29].

In approximately 13% of kidney cancer patients, genetic alterations in TSC1, PIK3A, or MET can be identified. While targeting the PI3K/mTOR pathway has demonstrated success in treating other cancers, such as breast cancer, it is important to note that in kidney cancer, having these alterations in the pathway is not currently a reliable predictor of how patients will respond to drugs that target it [6].

In contrast, MET is considered a more promising therapeutic target because multiple drugs can effectively inhibit this signalling pathway. Combining immunotherapy with anti-MET treatments, like cabozantinib, has shown encouraging and favourable results. However, it is worth noting that detecting the alteration is not an essential prerequisite for initiating first-line treatment [30].

Papillary kidney cancer may be characterized by activating mutations of MET [31]. Therapy with MET inhibitors in this type of neoplasm has manifested with very variable responses to therapy it was until recently; a comparison of different drugs in a phase two clinical trial positioned cabozantinib as the best alternative for patients with papillary kidney cancer due to its incidence of MET mutation [32].

Other biomarkers that may be involved in the prognosis of kidney cancer include survivin (BIRC5), XIAP, MCL-1, HIF1α, HIF2α, NRF2, MDM2, MDM4, TP5/p53, KRAS, and AKT [10].

Bladder Cancer

In recent years, there have been notable additions to the treatment options available for bladder cancer. However, we still lack reliable biomarkers to comprehensively determine prognosis and predict how patients respond to these treatments. The approval of various anti-PD-1 and PD-L1 immunotherapies for advanced bladder cancer treatment has underscored the importance of PD-L1 positivity as a response indicator, particularly in patients who cannot receive cisplatin. Multiple studies have confirmed the significance of PD-L1 positivity in both first and second-line treatments, showcasing the durability and depth of response [1].

The emergence of FGFR3-mutant urothelial bladder cancer has become noteworthy for patients who may initially appear resistant to immunotherapy. Erdafitinib, a targeted therapy, has demonstrated effectiveness in this context and is relevant for approximately 20% of cases [2].

Other biomarkers, such as nectin-4 and TROP-2, are the therapeutic targets of new conjugated antibodies (Enfortumab Vedotin and Sacituzumab Govitecan, respectively) for the treatment of advanced urothelial cancer; however, the measurement of both biomarkers is not recommended, because both biomarkers are intrinsically present in >90% of tumours, and their absence does not seem to confer prediction in treatment.

Looking to the future, through genetic sequencing, different research groups have divided bladder urothelial cancer into intrinsic molecular subtypes, and important differences have been observed in oncological outcomes in these subgroups. However, prospective evidence still needs to be improved to use them routinely.

Finally, other biomarkers, such as ERCC2, RB1, FANCC, and AT, have been investigated by genetic sequencing as predictive of response to treatment in early stages, and their clinical applicability is currently under discussion.

Many new therapies have recently been added to the treatment arsenal for bladder cancer. However, biomarkers are still lacking to determine the prognosis and predict treatment response fully. The approval of different anti-PD-1 and PD-L1 immunotherapies for the treatment of advanced bladder cancer has shown that the durability and depth of the response, especially in patients ineligible for cisplatin, PD-L1 positivity in these patients is considered a response marker in multiple studies in the first and second line of treatment [33-37].

In some cases where patients might not initially respond well to immunotherapy, bladder urothelial cancer with an FGFR3 mutation has gained significance. Using erdafitinib has demonstrated remarkable effectiveness and applies to approximately 20% of cases [38, 40].

Additionally, there are other biomarkers, such as nectin-4 and TROP-2, that serve as therapeutic targets for new antibody-conjugate treatments like Enfortumab Vedotin and Sacituzumab Govitecan in advanced urothelial cancer. However, accurately measuring both biomarkers remains a challenge. It is primarily because this type of cancer inherently exhibits both biomarkers in over 90% of tumours, and their absence does not appear to provide predictive value for treatment outcomes.

Looking ahead, genetic sequencing has enabled various research groups to categorize bladder urothelial cancer into distinct intrinsic molecular subtypes. These subtypes have shown substantial differences in oncological outcomes. However, it is important to note that there still needs to be more prospective evidence to support their routine clinical use [39, 40].

Finally, genetic sequencing has investigated other biomarkers as predictive markers of treatment response in the early stages. However, their clinical applicability is currently under discussion. These biomarkers include ERCC2, RB1, FANCC, and AT [38-40].

References

[1] American Cancer Society. *Cancer Facts & Figures* 2022.

[2] Pal M, Muinao T, Boruah HPD, Mahindroo N. Current advances in prognostic and diagnostic biomarkers for solid cancers: Detection techniques and future challenges. Vol. 146, *Biomedicine and Pharmacotherapy*. Elsevier Masson s.r.l.; 2022.

[3] Ilic D, Djulbegovic M, Jung JH, Hwang EC, Zhou Q, Cleves A, et al. Prostate cancer screening with prostate-specific antigen (PSA) test: A systematic review and meta-analysis. *BMJ (Online)*. 2018;362.

[4] Maruvada P, Wang W, Wagner PD, Srivastava S. *Biomarkers in molecular medicine: cancer detection and diagnosis*. 2005.

[5] Tondini C, Ciruelos E, Burstein HJ, Bonnefoi HR, Bellet M, Martino S, et al. Tailoring Adjuvant Endocrine Therapy for Premenopausal Breast Cancer. 2018;

[6] Dy GK, Nesline MK, Papanicolau-Sengos A, Depietro P, Levea CM, Early A, et al. Treatment recommendations to cancer patients in the context of FDA guidance for next-generation sequencing. *BMC Med Inform Decis Mak*. 2019 Jan 18;19(1).

[7] Tappia PS, Ramjiawan B. Biomarkers for Early Detection of Cancer: Molecular Aspects. *Int J Mol Sci*. 2023 Mar 9;24(6):5272.

[8] World Health Organization. Assessing national capacity for the prevention and control of noncommunicable diseases. 2019.

[9] Palazzo AF, Lee ES. Non-coding RNA: What is functional and what is junk? *Front Genet*. 2015;5(JAN).

[10] Yang M, Liu R, Sheng J, Liao J, Wang Y, Pan E, et al. Differential expression profiles of microRNAs as potential biomarkers for the early diagnosis of oesophagal squamous cell carcinoma. *Oncol Rep*. 2013 Jan;29(1):169–76.

[11] Wang WT, Chen YQ. Circulating miRNAs in cancer: From detection to therapy. Vol. 7, Journal of Hematology and Oncology. *BioMed Central Ltd*.; 2014.

[12] Gayosso-Gómez LV, Ortiz-Quintero B. Circulating microRNAs in blood and other body fluids as biomarkers for diagnosis, prognosis, and therapy response in lung cancer. *Diagnostics*. 2021 Mar 1;11(3).

[13] Sung H, Ferlay J, Siegel RL, Laversanne M, Soerjomataram I, Jemal A, et al. Global Cancer Statistics 2020: GLOBOCAN Estimates of Incidence and Mortality Worldwide for 36 Cancers in 185 Countries. *CA Cancer J Clin*. 2021 May;71(3):209–49.

[14] Yaxiong Z, Jin S, Shiyang K. Patients with Exon 19 Deletion Were Associated with Longer Progression-Free Survival Compared to Those with L858R Mutation after First-Line EGFR-TKIs for Advanced Non-Small Cell Lung Cancer: A Meta-Analysis. *PLoS One*. 2014 Mar 1;9(9).

[15] Oxnard GR, Thress KS, Alden RS, Lawrance R, Paweletz CP, Cantarini M, et al. Association between plasma genotyping and treatment outcomes with osimertinib (AZD9291) in advanced non-small-cell lung cancer. *Journal of Clinical Oncology*. 2016 Oct 1;34(28):3375–82.

[16] Chabon JJ, Simmons AD, Lovejoy AF, Esfahani MS, Newman AM, Haringsma HJ, et al. Circulating tumour DNA profiling reveals heterogeneity of EGFR inhibitor resistance mechanisms in lung cancer patients. *Nat Commun*. 2016 Jun 10;7.

[17] Soda M, Choi YL, Enomoto M, Takada S, Yamashita Y, Ishikawa S, et al. Identification of the transforming EML4-ALK fusion gene in non-small-cell lung cancer. *Nature*. 2007 Aug 2;448(7153):561–6.

[18] Shaw AT, Kim DW, Mehra R, Tan DSW, Felip E, Chow LQM, et al. Ceritinib in ALK -Rearranged Non–Small-Cell Lung Cancer. *New England Journal of Medicine*. 2014 Mar 27;370(13):1189–97.

[19] Camidge DR, Kim HR, Ahn MJ, Yang JCH, Han JY, Lee JS, et al. Brigatinib versus Crizotinib in ALK -Positive Non–Small-Cell Lung Cancer. *New England Journal of Medicine*. 2018 Nov 22;379(21):2027–39.

[20] Lindeman NI, Cagle PT, Aisner DL, Arcila ME, Beasley MB, Bernicker EH, et al. Updated molecular testing guidelines for selecting lung cancer patients for treatment with targeted tyrosine kinase inhibitors guidelines from the College of American Pathologists, the International Association for the Study of Lung Cancer, and the Association for Molecular Pathology. In: *Archives of Pathology and Laboratory Medicine*. College of American Pathologists; 2018. p. 321–46.

[21] Lindeman NI, Cagle PT, Beasley MB, Chitale DA, Dacic S, Giaccone G, et al. Molecular testing guideline for selecting lung cancer patients for EGFR and ALK tyrosine kinase inhibitors: Guideline from the College of American Pathologists, International Association for the study of lung cancer, and Association for Molecular Pathology. *Arch Pathol Lab Med*. 2013 Jun;137(6):828–60.

[22] Lim SM, Syn NL, Cho BC, Soo RA. Acquired resistance to EGFR targeted therapy in non-small cell lung cancer: Mechanisms and therapeutic strategies. Vol. 65, *Cancer Treatment Reviews*. W.B. Saunders Ltd; 2018. p. 1–10.

[23] Tamminga M, De Wit S, Hiltermann TJN, Timens W, Schuuring E, Terstappen LWMM, et al. Circulating tumour cells in advanced non-small cell lung cancer patients are associated with worse tumour response to checkpoint inhibitors. *J Immunother Cancer*. 2019 Jul 10;7(1).

[24] Kristina Gregory N, Miranda Hughes O, Aisner DL, Akerley W, Bauman JR, Bruno DS, et al. NCCN Guidelines Version 3.*2023 Non-Small Cell Lung Cancer Continue NCCN Guidelines Panel Disclosures [Internet]*. 2023. Available from: https://www.nccn.org/home/member.

[25] Siegel RL, Miller KD, Wagle NS, Jemal A. Cancer statistics, 2023. *CA Cancer J Clin*. 2023;73(1):17.

[26] Heng DY, Xie W, Regan MM, Harshman LC, Bjarnason GA, Vaishampayan UN, et al. External validation and comparison with other models of the International Metastatic Renal-Cell Carcinoma Database Consortium prognostic model: a population-based study. *Lancet Oncol*. 2013;14(2):141-8.

[27] Tannir NM, McDermott DF, Escudier B, Hammers HJ, Aren OR, Plimack ER, et al. Overall survival and independent review of response in CheckMate 214 with 42-month follow-up: First-line nivolumab + ipilimumab (N+I) versus sunitinib (S) in patients (pts) with advanced renal cell carcinoma (aRCC). *Journal of Clinical Oncology*. 2020;38(6_suppl):609.

[28] Terry S, Dalban C, Rioux-Leclercq N, Adam J, Meylan M, Buart S, et al. Association of AXL and PD-L1 Expression with Clinical Outcomes in Patients with

Advanced Renal Cell Carcinoma Treated with PD-1 Blockade. *Clin Cancer Res.* 2021;27(24):6749-60.

[29] Xu W, Atkins MB, McDermott DF. Checkpoint inhibitor immunotherapy in kidney cancer. *Nat Rev Urol.* 2020;17(3):137-50.

[30] Motzer RJ, Hutson TE, Glen H, Michaelson MD, Molina A, Eisen T, et al. Lenvatinib, everolimus, and the combination in patients with metastatic renal cell carcinoma: a randomised, phase 2, open-label, multicentre trial. *Lancet Oncol.* 2015;16(15):1473-82.

[31] Choueiri TK, Powles T, Burotto M, Escudier B, Bourlon MT, Zurawski B, et al. Nivolumab plus Cabozantinib versus Sunitinib for Advanced Renal-Cell Carcinoma. *N Engl J Med.* 2021;384(9):829-41.

[32] Albiges L, Guegan J, Le Formal A, Verkarre V, Rioux-Leclercq N, Sibony M, et al. MET is a potential target across all papillary renal cell carcinomas: result from a large molecular study of pRCC with CGH array and matching gene expression array. *Clin Cancer Res.* 2014;20(13):3411-21.

[33] Pal SK, Tangen C, Thompson IM, Jr., Balzer-Haas N, George DJ, Heng DYC, et al. A comparison of sunitinib with cabozantinib, crizotinib, and savolitinib for treatment of advanced papillary renal cell carcinoma: a randomised, open-label, phase 2 trial. *Lancet.* 2021;397(10275):695-703.

[34] Li F, Aljahdali IAM, Zhang R, Nastiuk KL, Krolewski JJ, Ling X. Kidney cancer biomarkers and targets for therapeutics: survivin (BIRC5), XIAP, MCL-1, HIF1α, HIF2α, NRF2, MDM2, MDM4, p53, KRAS and AKT in renal cell carcinoma. *J Exp Clin Cancer Res.* 2021;40(1):254.

[35] Balar AV, Castellano D, O'Donnell PH, Grivas P, Vuky J, Powles T, et al. First-line pembrolizumab in cisplatin-ineligible patients with locally advanced and unresectable or metastatic urothelial cancer (KEYNOTE-052): a multicentre, single-arm, phase 2 study. *Lancet Oncol.* 2017;18(11):1483-92.

[36] Balar AV, Galsky MD, Rosenberg JE, Powles T, Petrylak DP, Bellmunt J, et al. Atezolizumab as first-line treatment in cisplatin-ineligible patients with locally advanced and metastatic urothelial carcinoma: a single-arm, multicentre, phase 2 trial. *Lancet.* 2017;389(10064):67-76.

[37] Rosenberg JE, Hoffman-Censits J, Powles T, van der Heijden MS, Balar AV, Necchi A, et al. Atezolizumab in patients with locally advanced and metastatic urothelial carcinoma who have progressed following treatment with platinum-based chemotherapy: a single-arm, multicentre, phase 2 trial. *Lancet.* 2016;387(10031):1909-20.

[38] Baylin SB, Jones PA. Epigenetic determinants of cancer. *Cold Spring Harb Perspect Biol.* 2016;8(9):a019505. doi:10.1101/cshperspect.a019505.

[39] Melo SA, Esteller M. Epigenetics in cancer: Friends or foes? *Curr Opin Genet Dev.* 2017;42:1-3. doi:10.1016/j.gde.2017.01.006.

[40] Rauschert S, Raiss C, Wang Z, et al. Epigenetic biomarker screening by FLIM-FRET for precision medicine in bladder cancer. *Cancer Res.* 2020;80(2):363-375. doi:10.1158/0008-5472.CAN-19.

Chapter 5

Classification and Identification of Gene Markers in the Medulloblastoma Subgroup by Implementing the Support Vector Machine

Lalu Bayu Dwi Cahyo[1]
and Rohmatul Fajriyah[2,*]

[1]PT Semesta Integrasi Digital, Business Unit Talentics, Indonesia
[2]Master Program in Statistics, Department Statistics, Universitas Islam Indonesia, Yogyakarta, Indonesia

Abstract

Medulloblastoma is a heterogeneous group of malignant tumours of the central nerve system (CNS). It is relatively rare; 18%-20% of all cancerous pediatric brain tumours and 70% of all pediatric medulloblastomas are diagnosed in children under age 10. Medulloblastoma has four subgroups: WNT (wingless), SHH(sonic hedgehog), Subgroup 3, and Subgroup 4. We implement a Support Vector Machine to classify and identify the group's gene markers. The analysis shows that the SVM model has a prediction accuracy of 0.93 in the training data set and a multiclass accuracy of 0.9896 with an AUC of 0.938 in the testing data set. The SVM model has an outstanding performance. We chose ten gene markers based on the most important ones. The gene names are ribosomal protein L18, L18a, S2, S3, S14, S15, S17, S18, S19, and lateral stalk subunit P1.

Keywords: medulloblastoma, CNS, support vector machine, gene markers, ribosomal protein

---

[*] Corresponding Author's Email: 966110101@uii.ac.id.

In: A Closer Look at Cancer Biomarkers
Editor: Arli Aditya Parikesit
ISBN: 979-8-89113-497-3
© 2024 Nova Science Publishers, Inc.

1. Introduction

Technological developments in the 21st-century era of globalization are followed by an explosion of large amounts of data, or what is often known as big data. Big Data is a technology system introduced to overcome the 'information explosion' and the growing ecosystem of mobile device users and internet data. Big data has three terms, namely volume, variety, and velocity. Volume relates to the size of the data storage media, which is very large or unlimited; variety means the type or type of data that can be accommodated, and velocity can be interpreted as the processing speed (Perry, 2017).

Data development occurs in almost all science fields, including molecular biology, known as bioinformatics. Bioinformatics is an application of science that studies the application of computer science to managing and analyzing biological information. Bioinformatics includes the application of statistical and informatics methods to solve biological problems (Attwood, 1999).

Discussion of bioinformatics will include sequencing and microarrays (microchips). The official website of the American National Center for Biotechnology Information (NCBI) defines a microarray as the hybridization of a nucleic acid sample (target) to a set of large, solidly attached oligonucleotide probes for sequence determination or for detecting variations in gene sequence or expression or for mapping gene.

The existence of a microarray, which is a sequencing of an organism's data, certainly has a large amount of data and dimensions following the previous explanation. The microarray contains information from a collection of probes from a gene.

One of these implementations is storing gene data of patients who have contracted brain cancer in children, namely Medulloblastoma. Medulloblastoma is a heterogeneous group of malignant central nervous system (CNS) tumours affecting young males. Based on the e-book entitled Medulloblastoma, released by ABTA (American Brain Tumor Association) in 2015, Medulloblastoma is relatively rare and aggressive, characterized by a metastatic tendency, accounting for less than 2% of all primary brain tumours (tumours that start in the brain or on its surface), between 18% -20% of all brain tumours that affect children. Medulloblastoma is the most common malignant brain tumour in children aged four years and under and the second most common in children aged 5-14 years, and 70% of sufferers of Medulloblastoma are detected at the age of 10 years and below.

Medulloblastoma is formed due to errors in cell functions that control cell growth and death. The reason this happens still needs to be understood.

However, scientists are making significant progress in understanding what happens inside these cells that turn normal brain cells into cancerous growths. These changes are identified in genes and chromosomes (DNA cells) that play a role in their development.

Robinson et al. (2012) and Morfuace et al. (2015) conducted data collection on 76 young patients infected with Medulloblastoma with the title "Novel mutations target distinct subgroups of medulloblastoma. "Their research classifies patients into four classes: WNT (wingless), SHH (sonic hedgehog), Group 3, and Group 4.

Recent developments in the molecular biology of Medulloblastoma indicate that the classification of embryonic tumours based solely on histological and clinical criteria needs to be revised. A better understanding of growth control mechanisms in the development and progression of Medulloblastoma will enable better classification, improving existing therapies, and developing new therapeutic approaches (Rossi et al., 2008).

Based on those mentioned above in this paper, we are interested in building a classification model for Medulloblastoma. This paper is organized as follows: the first section is about the introduction, then the literature review, the statistical method used in the analysis, results, and discussion, and the final section is the conclusion and remarks.

2. Literature Review

Aprijani (2004), in a book entitled "Bioinformatics: Development, Discipline of Science and Its Application in Indonesia," explains that bioinformatics combines molecular biology disciplines, mathematics, and information engineering. It was concluded that bioinformatics is an application of computation and data analysis on molecular biology data. Bioinformatics has the potential to develop because it is multi-disciplinary, but bioinformatics in Indonesia has yet to be popular in the community.

Lesk (2011) described that bioinformatics is a cross-section of knowledge that refers to biological data and information collection, distribution, and analysis techniques to support a combination of scientific research, including biomedicine. Developing efficient algorithms for measuring sequence similarity is the goal of bioinformatics. The Needleman-Wunsch algorithm based on dynamic programming guarantees to find the optimal alignment of sequence pairs. The algorithm divides a big problem (complete sequence) into a series of more minor problems (short sequence segment) and uses smaller problem solutions to build big problem solutions. Similarities within sequences are assessed in a matrix, and the algorithm makes it possible to detect gaps in the alignment of the sequences.

Cahyo (2017) stated that Boser, Guyon, and Vapnik developed the Support Vector Machine (SVM), first presented in 1992 at the Annual Workshop on Computational Learning Theory. The basic concept of SVM is a harmonious combination of computational theories that existed decades before, such as margin hyperplane and kernel. There had never been an attempt to assemble these components until 1992.

An application of SVM in bioinformatics research can be seen in Brown (1999), who concluded that SVM can accurately classify genes into functional categories and make predictions to identify the function of unannotated yeast genes. Paper of Nugroho (2003), Chicco (2012), Alshamlan et al. (2013), and Bhat (2017) also described the application of SVM in bioinformatics, especially the analysis of gene expression obtained from microarray experiments on cancer patients.

Furey et al. (2000) conducted research entitled "Support Vector Machine Classification and Validation of Cancer Tissue Samples Using Microarray Expression Data. "In their research, the methods of SVM and perceptron are used. Based on this research, it was found that SVM can classify tissue and cell types, just like the perceptron algorithm. In addition, SVM can also be used to identify mislabeled data. In this study, a simple kernel was applied.

Northcott (2014) conducted a Medulloblastoma study comprising four distinct molecular variants. Based on his research, brain tumours are the leading cause of cancer-related death in children, and Medulloblastoma is the most malignant brain tumour in children. Based on the gene expression and DNA aberrations of 103 medulloblastoma patients and applying statistical methods (ANOVA, NMF, PCA, SubMap, path analysis, and hierarchical clustering), identified four nonoverlapping molecular variant groups, namely WNT, SHH, group C, and group D.

Upadhyay (2014) stated that the results are more significant in children with Medulloblastoma when treated with radical surgical excision and adjuvant therapy in the long term. The best and worst results from the respective treatment were in the WNT pathway and non-WNT/non-SHH groups; for children in the SHH group, the results would be between the two. Studies in India based on molecular subtyping prove that molecular subtyping is feasible, cost-effective, and value-added in prognosticating outcomes for children with Medulloblastoma.

In microarray cancer research, the objectives and methods are used for gene finding, class discovery, and class prediction (Alshamlan, 2013). Based on his research, Choi (2023) concluded that it is necessary to incorporate genetic findings into the standard of care, and clinical trials that reflect this need to be conducted.

3. Basic Concept

3.1. DNA and Gene Expression (Fajriyah, 2021)

DNA is a nucleic acid with a sugar component of deoxyribose, and the base components are A, C, G, and T. The deoxyribose sugar consists of 5 carbons and oxygen in a ring, and the carbons are numbered 5', 4', 3', 2', and 1'. The ' is read as prime, a naming convention that means to the carbons in the deoxyribose ring, not the carbons of the base.

DNA is a double helix with two nucleotide chains with a linear sugar (S) and phosphate (P) backbone. In this form, the direction of the nucleotides in one strand is opposite to their direction in the other. The ends of DNA strands are called the 5 'and 3 'ends. It refers to the locations of carbons on the pentose sugars. The double helix is formed due to the hydrogen bonding between base pairs. The bases on one strand are paired with the bases on another strand, according to Watson- Crick base pairing rules, where A specifically pairs with T, and C will pair with G (Amaratunga & Cabrera, 2004; Draghici, 2003; Zhang, 2006). It is repeated millions or billions of times throughout a genome. The order of As, Ts, Cs, and Gs dictates whether an organism is human or another species, such as yeast, rice, or fruit flies.

DNA in each human cell is packaged into 46 chromosomes and arranged into 23 pairs. Each chromosome is a physically separate molecule of DNA that ranges in length from about 50 million to 250 million base pairs (Amaratunga & Cabrera, 2004). Each chromosome contains many genes, the basic physical and functional units of heredity for an organism (Lee, 2006). The structure at the end of the chromosome, an area of highly repetitive DNA sequences, is called a telomere.

An RNA is a nucleic acid with the sugar component of ribose (has an -OH at the 2 'C position, whereas the DNA sugar has an -H at that position), and the base component contains base uracil instead of thymine. It is a single-stranded. Genes are specific sequences of bases that encode instructions for making proteins or RNA molecules (Amaratunga & Cabrera, 2004; Draghici, 2003; Lee, 2006; Zhang, 2006). The process whereby a gene transfers its genetic code information from DNA into protein is called gene expression.

Firstly, the DNA double helix splits and develops a condition where one strand of the DNA acts as a template where the complementary messenger ribonucleic acid (mRNA) is formed. The mRNA strand then separates. The sequence bases of mRNA are then converted into proteins through the translation step. All the processes are formulated in a central dogma of molecular biology (Amaratunga & Cabrera, 2004).

3.2. Microarrays

Microarrays have been widely used in biomedical research. It is a tool designed to measure the expression levels of thousands of genes in a disease or cell type. (Bolstad, 2004). The cells in the human body contain identical genetic material, but the same genes are not active in every cell (Fajriyah, 2021). Some genes are active or appear only when needed. Microarray technology determines whether the gene is active or not in a cell. Especially in cells with different conditions, examples come from tissues such as regular or cancer tissues.

To determine which genes are turned on and which are turned off in a given cell, a researcher must conduct microarray experiments (Fajriyah, 2021).

1. The mRNA molecules present in that cell are extracted, isolated, and purified by following the specific protocol based on the company of the chosen technology.
2. The researcher labels each mRNA molecule using a reverse transcriptase enzyme (RT). This process will generate a complementary oligonucleotide to the mRNA. During that process, fluorescent nucleotides are attached to the mRNA.
3. The researcher places the labelled mRNAs onto a DNA microarray slide. The labelled mRNAs representing mRNAs in the cell will then hybridize -or bind- to their synthetic complementary DNA or oligonucleotides attached to the microarray slide.
4. The researcher then uses a scanner to measure the fluorescent intensity for each feature on the microarray slide. If a particular gene is very active in a given cell, it produces many mRNA molecules.

Therefore, the hybridization process will generate very bright fluorescence. Less active genes produce fewer mRNAs and will produce dimmer fluorescence. If there is no fluorescence, none of the messenger molecules has hybridized to the target on the microarray slide, indicating that the gene is inactive. The intensity value of the scanned image of the microarray slide after hybridization, washing, and staining measures the gene expression were measured accordingly.

There are two types of microarray technologies: oligonucleotide and sequencing. Oligonucleotide DNA microarrays are divided into two subgroups: long oligonucleotide arrays, whose probes consist of 60-mer or 50-mer DNA sequences (e.g., Illumina Beadarray), and short oligonucleotide arrays that use 25-mer (e.g., Affymetrix GeneChip) or 30-mer of probe sequence design. Affymetrix GeneChip uses technology like computer silicon chips. Affymetrix silicon material is protected by sealing and applying a photolithographic process to control oligonucleotide synthesis on the glass/plastic surface. Probe design matches different genes using 25-mer oligonucleotide-specific genes, specifically, a probe set formed with 11 to 20 different probe pairs. The probe pair designs are mismatch (MM) and perfect match(PM) probes. The MM probe was used to control for nonspecific binding during hybridization. One of the unique features of the GeneChip array is that each pair of probes is attached to a predetermined location on the surface of the array (Bolstad, 2004).

3.3. Pre-Processing

One step in microarray data analysis is pre-processing. It was the first step and the most important one. This step ensures that the data is valid and reliable such that the conclusion from the analysis is trustworthy, see Fajriyah (2021). Different steps are applied in the pre-processing of microarray data. It generally includes background correction, normalization, probe correction, and summarization.

Background correction generally refers to fixed background noise and processing effects. Normalization is the process of removing unwanted non-biological endings between chips in a microarray experiment. The summarization is a process to produce the gene expression value.

3.4. Filtering

Filtering is a process to select some probes to be excluded or excluded in the analysis. As Bourgon (2010) stated, filtering removes features that show several minor variants or data discrepancies consistently across samples, which can be helpful in further analysis.

There are two types of filtering: specific and nonspecific filtering. In this paper, we used the *gene-filter* R package to filter. The function *nsFilter* is a one-stop-shop option for various filtering options (removal) features from the expression set. The function shows if Entrez is used in filtering (a database that stores related genes). The function removes dupEntrez, which removes the duplicate Entrez ID and the genes where the variance is less than 0.5. The data obtained after this process has a lower dimension than the original one.

The specific filtering is then applied to remove genes not differentially expressed across 4 group samples. It was done by implementing the ANOVA and *gene-filter* functions.

3.6. Support Vector Machine

SVM (support vector machine) in machine learning is also known as a support vector network, a supervised method for learning algorithms for analyzing data patterns. It is used for classification and regression (Mohammed et al., 2017).

When Vapnik first introduced the time, SVM could only classify data into two classes (binary classification). Further research on developing SVM to classify data with more than two classes continues. An option is to implement multiclass SVM by combining several binary SVMs or all data consisting of several classes into an optimization problem. The second approach is that the optimization problems to be solved are much more complicated.

SVM uses the dot product function in binary classes to find the best hyperplane, a separator for two classes in the input space (Nugroho, 2003).

For the multiclass SVM, two methods are commonly used, namely the "one-against-all" and the "one-against-one" methods (Liu and Xheng (2005), Milgram et al. (2006)). The binary SVM model is built using *the one-against-all* method, k where k is the number of classes. For *the one-against-one* method, the $(k(k-1)/2)$ binary classification models are built (k, the number of classes). Each classification model is trained on data from two classes. There are several methods for conducting tests after the entire $(k(k-1)/2)$

classification model has been built. One is the voting method, where the majority will be voted as the final result.

3.8. ROC (Receiver Operating Characteristics) curve

The ROC (Receiver Operating Characteristic) curve is a method that can be used to assess the performance of a test (Bolstad, 2004). The test is depicted in a curve with the vertical axis representing the accurate positive level (sensitivity). It means that a class is predicted to enter the positive class, and the results are correct. The horizontal axis label is a false positive (1-sensitivity) level, meaning that the predicted data class enters the positive class, and the result is wrong. This method will give 100% results if nothing goes wrong.

Although Chicco and Jurman (2023) have recently proposed using the Matthews correlation coefficient (MCC) to replace the ROC, in this paper, we still use the ROC to assess the multiclass classification.

4. Results and Discussion

4.1. Statistical Descriptive

This paper uses the GSE37418 data set based on Robinson et al. (2012) and Morfuace (2015). It is a collection of gene expression samples from pediatric medulloblastoma patients. There are 76 patients with Medulloblastoma with different characteristics such as ethnicity, sex, age, and medulloblastoma type. Upadhyay (2014) divided Medulloblastoma into four subtypes, and this GSE37418 data has 4 of the same subtypes as Upadhyay mentioned, and the remaining three patients had no subtypes. Therefore, the data used in this study were 73 patients belonging to 4 subtypes, namely WNT, SHH, Subgroup 3, and Subgroup 4.

Figure 1 shows that the classes are imbalanced, where 53%, 22%, 14%, and 11% of patients, respectively, belong to subgroup 4, subgroup 3, SHH, and WNT. Each group will get different treatment for the recuperation process. Figure 2 elicits the gender distribution of the data set.

There were more male patients in this sample compared to female patients. Most patients are nine years old; this is in line with what ABTA has written, which is that patients with Medulloblastoma are more likely children under ten years old.

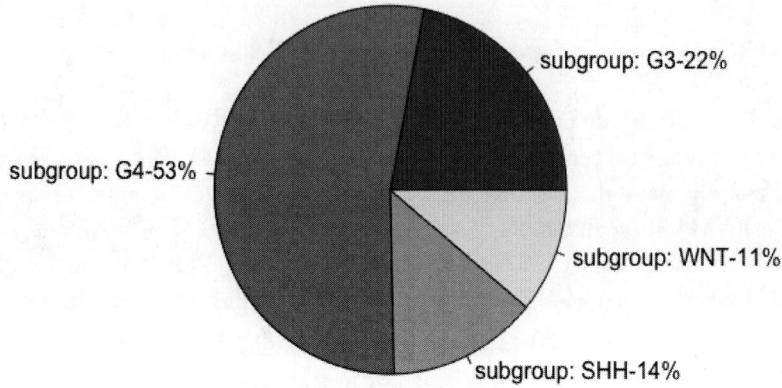

Figure 1. Medulloblastoma type in the GSE37418 data set.

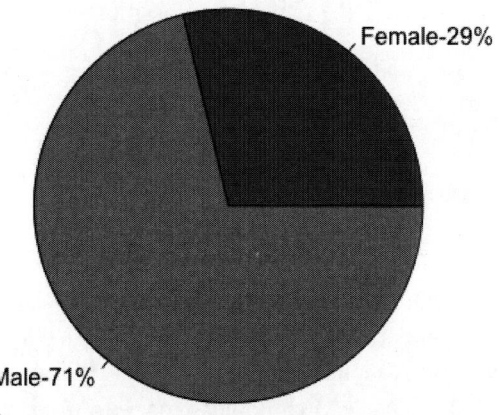

Figure 2. Medulloblastoma patient's gender in the GSE37418 data set.

Figure 3 shows the number of each patient ethnicity. The white ethnicity is the most (43/73) because the sample collection was carried out in America, where the majority of the population is white, 13/73 are from Hispanic, 6/73 from Asia, 4/ from Indian and Black ethnicity, three others, and one patient from Pacific Islander ethnicity.

In the study, pre-processing is done using the *three-step* function from the affyPLM package. The background correction method used is RMA.2, the normalization method used is quantile, and the summarization method is median.

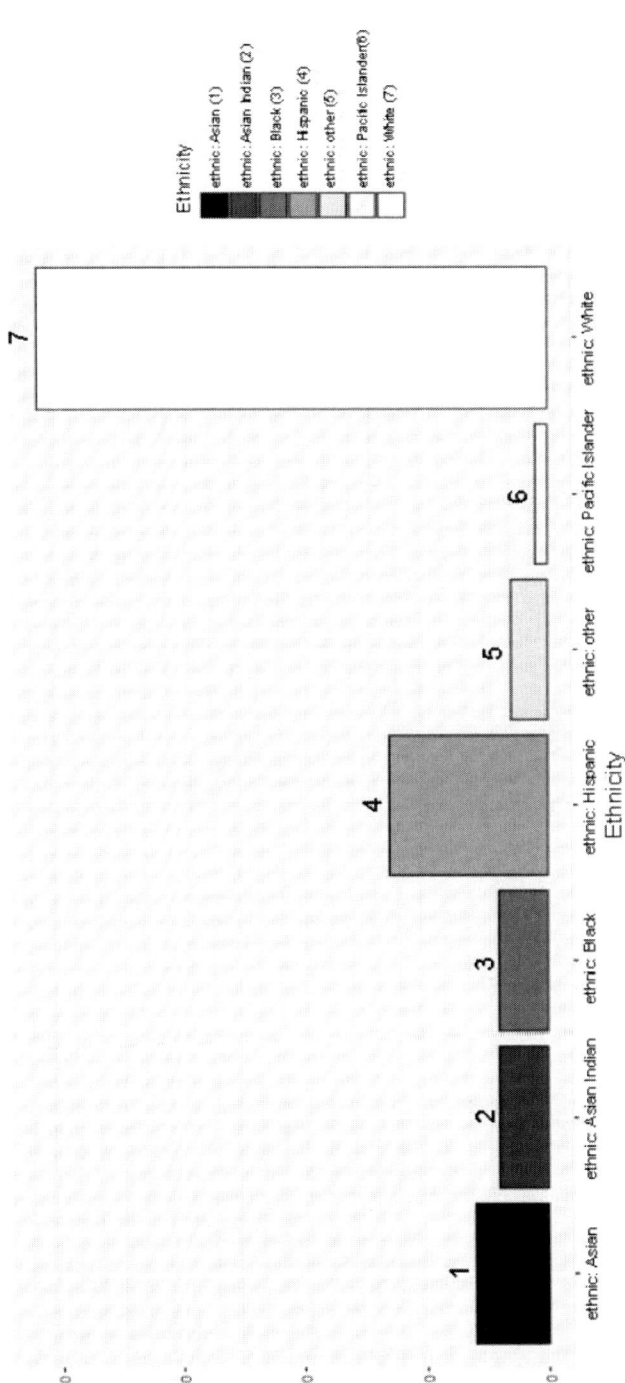

Figure 3. Ethnicity for *Medulloblastoma* GSE37418 data set.

For the nonspecific filtering, the *nsFilter* function is used here. The initial genes are 54,675; after this filtering, it is reduced to 10,251. Then, we applied the specific filtering using the *gene-filter* function with the ANOVA method. Because there are four groups, the genes are further reduced to 5,226. These 5,226 genes are used in the classification data analysis by using SVM.

4.2. Analysis

The data classification uses 2 data sets, namely training and testing data sets, with a proportion of 80% (58 samples) and 20% (15 samples) data sets. The preliminary study compares the costs between 0.1, 0.01, 0.001, 1, 10, and 100. Then, among these values, the best cost for the data set is 0.1. Therefore, a cost of 0.1 is used to build the model on the training data set.

The confusion matrix evaluates the model generated using the training data (Chin et al., 2010). The confusion matrix shows that each prediction based on the model on the training data produces a classification according to the class; each subgroup does not give the wrong classification. The prediction obtained with the test data has an accuracy of 0.93. It contains one error only where the patient is predicted to be classified as subgroup G4. The patient is classified as subgroup G3. The model's results based on the confusion matrix are good, but ROC is used to test further validation.

Table 1. The most important variables based on their weights

No	Genes (Probes id)	weight
1	212433_x_at	0.0094
2	201049_s_at	0.0093
3	200869_at	0.0091
4	213414_s_at	0.0091
5	200022_at	0.0091
6	200819_s_at	0.0091
7	208692_at	0.0091
8	201665_x_at	0.0090
9	200763_s_at	0.0090
10	208645_s_at	0.0090

Based on the computation, the multiclass AUC value is 0.9583, which can be considered high because the maximum value is 1. A high AUC value indicates that the model obtained is good and can be used to predict the classification.

We know that after the last filtering, we have 5226 genes, which are used to model the classification for the medulloblastoma classification. We built the model already, and it has good accuracy. Further analysis, we would like to know which genes among 5226 are the most important to classify the data. The ten essential variables in the SVM model are in Table 1. These genes can be considered as the gene markers of the medulloblastoma class.

Table 2. Gene ontology for the most important genes

PROBEID	SYMBOL	GENE NAME	ENTREZID	ONTOLOGY
212433_x_at	RPS2	ribosomal protein S2	6187	BP
212433_x_at	RPS2	ribosomal protein S2	6187	CC
212433_x_at	RPS2	ribosomal protein S2	6187	MF
201049_s_at	RPS18	ribosomal protein S18	6222	BP
201049_s_at	RPS18	ribosomal protein S18	6222	CC
201049_s_at	RPS18	ribosomal protein S18	6222	MF
200869_at	RPL18A	ribosomal protein L18a	6142	BP
PROBEID	SYMBOL	GENE NAME	ENTREZID	ONTOLOGY
200869_at	RPL18A	ribosomal protein L18a	6142	CC
200869_at	RPL18A	ribosomal protein L18a	6142	MF
213414_s_at	RPS19	ribosomal protein S19	6223	BP
213414_s_at	RPS19	ribosomal protein S19	6223	CC
213414_s_at	RPS19	ribosomal protein S19	6223	MF
200022_at	RPL18	ribosomal protein L18	6141	BP
200022_at	RPL18	ribosomal protein L18	6141	CC
200022_at	RPL18	ribosomal protein L18	6141	MF
200819_s_at	RPS15	ribosomal protein S15	6209	BP
200819_s_at	RPS15	ribosomal protein S15	6209	CC
200819_s_at	RPS15	ribosomal protein S15	6209	MF
208692_at	RPS3	ribosomal protein S3	6188	BP
208692_at	RPS3	ribosomal protein S3	6188	CC
208692_at	RPS3	ribosomal protein S3	6188	MF
201665_x_at	RPS17	ribosomal protein S17	6218	BP
201665_x_at	RPS17	ribosomal protein S17	6218	CC
201665_x_at	RPS17	ribosomal protein S17	6218	MF
200763_s_at	RPLP1	ribosomal protein lateral stalk subunit P1	6176	BP
200763_s_at	RPLP1	ribosomal protein lateral stalk subunit P1	6176	CC
200763_s_at	RPLP1	ribosomal protein lateral stalk subunit P1	6176	MF
208645_s_at	RPS14	ribosomal protein S14	6208	BP
208645_s_at	RPS14	ribosomal protein S14	6208	CC
208645_s_at	RPS14	ribosomal protein S14	6208	MF

Table 2 shows the name of the gene from which the probe is derived and its gene ontology. Gene ontology (GO) is a framework for biological models.

GO is defined as a concept or class used to describe gene function and the relationship between the concepts. In GO, there are three functions, namely BP (biological process), MF (molecular function), and CC (Cellular Component).

Table 2 shows that the probe originates from the ribosomal protein gene and belongs to the three functions in GO. When we investigated until the 50th probes, we found that probes 225547_at and 225155_at are small nucleolar RNA host genes 6 and 5 and do not belong to any GO.

The multiple hypothesis testing and heatmap show that the ten genes are over-expressed in the SHH, WNT, and G3 and under-expressed in G4 medulloblastoma types. The enrichment and analysis could further be done to understand the gene-gene interactions regarding this disease.

Conclusion

The study showed that the classification model based on the SVM method has a prediction accuracy of 93.33% with a multiclass AUC value of 98.96%. The high accuracy indicates that the SVM model can predict the classification well.

The gene markers to classify medulloblastoma type are based on the ten highest weights of the importance variables. The gene names are *ribosomal protein* L18, L18a, S2, S3, S14, S15, S17, S18, S19, and *lateral stalk subunit P1*. All genes have their ontology known. As for genes with the IDs 225547_at and 225155_at, further analysis in the wet laboratory is needed to confirm whether both genes are the new gene markers for the medulloblastoma type. If they are, then it will affect the treatment approach for the disease, as Choi (2023) has highlighted.

References

ABTA, Medulloblastoma, 2015, http://www.abta.org/secure/medulloblastoma-brochure.pdf access May 15, 2023.

Alshamlan H. M., Badr G. H., Alohali Y. A. (2013). A Study of Cancer Microarray Gene Expression Profile: Objectives and Approaches London, U.K. *Proceeding of the World Congress on Engineering* 2013 Vol II pp. 1-6.

Aprijani D. A., and Elfaizi M. Abdushshomad, (2003), Bioinformatika: Perkembangan, Disiplin Ilmu dan Penerapannya di Indonesia, ftp://202.125.94.81/pub/linux/docs/v06/Kuliah/SistemOperasi/2003/50/Bioinformatika.pdf. Access May 15, 2023.

Amaratunga, A., and Cabrera J. (2004). Exploration and analysis of DNA microarray and protein array data. New Jersey: John Wiley & Sons.

Attwood, T. K., and Parry-Smith, D. J. (1999). Introduction to Bioinformatics, Harlow: Pearson Education.

Bhat, H. F., (2017). Evaluating SVM Algorithms for Bioinformatics Gene Expression Analysis. IJCSE. http://www.ijcse.net/docs/IJCSE17-06-02-023.pdf access May 15, 2023. 6:42-52.

Bolstad M. B. (2004). Low-level Analysis of High-density Oligonucleotide Array Data: Background, Normalization and Summarization .https://pdfs.semanticscholar.org/a0e2/3447 9d90b24f5 9791b3d52bbf2cb27d90acf.pdf. access May 15, 2023.

Bourgon R., Gentleman R., Huber W. Independent filtering increases detection power for high-throughput experiments. *Proc Natl Acad Sci U S A*. 2010 May 25;107(21):9546–51. doi: 10.1073/pnas.0914005107. Epub 2010 May 11. PMID: 20460310; PMCID: PMC2906865.

Brown M. P., Grundy W. N., Lin D., Cristianini N., Sugnet C. W., Furey T. S., Ares M. Jr, Haussler D. (2000). Knowledge-based analysis of microarray gene expression data using support vector machines. 4;97(1):262-7. doi: 10.1073/pnas.97.1.262. PMID: 10618406; PMCID: PMC26651.

Buehler L. K., and Rashidi, H. H. (2005). Bioinformatics Basic: Applications in biological science and medicine, Boca Raton, FL. CRC Press.

Cahyo, L. B. D. (2017). Implementasi Metode Support Vector machine untuk Melakukan Klasifikasi pada Data Bioinformatika, Skripsi, Prodi Statistika FMIPA UII, Yogyakarta.

Chicco D. (2012). *Support Vector Machines in Bioinformatics: A Survey.* http://www.DavideChicco.it. Access May 15, 2023.

Chicco D., Jurman G. The Matthews correlation coefficient (MCC) should replace the ROC AUC as the standard metric for assessing binary classification. *BioData Mining* 16, 4 (2023). https://doi.org/10.1186/s13040-023-00322-4.

Chin, W., Chang C., Lin, C. 2010. *A Practical Guide to Support Vector Classification.* Taiwan: Department of Computer Science National Taiwan University.

Choi, J. Y. (2023). Medulloblastoma: Current Perspective and Recent Advances, *Brain Tumor Research and Treatment*, 11(1), 28-38, doi: 10.14791/btrt.2022.0046.

Draghici, S. (2003). Data analysis tools for DNA microarrays. Florida: Chapman & Hall.

Fajriyah, R. (2021). Paper review: An overview of microarray technologies. *Bulletin of Applied Mathematics and Mathematics Education, 1*(1), 21–30.

Furey T. S., Duffy N., Cristianini N., Bednarski, D., Schummer, M. Dan Haussler D. Support Vector Machine Classification and Validation of Cancer Tissue Samples Using Microarray Expression Data. Bioinformatics. 2000, 16(10):906-914.

Liu Y. and Zheng Y. F., (2005). One-against-all multiclass SVM classification using reliability measures, *Proceedings. 2005 IEEE International Joint Conference on Neural Networks*, 2005., Montreal, Que., 2005, pp. 849-854 vol. 2, doi: 10.1109/IJCNN.2005.1555963.

Lee M. L. (2006). Analysis of microarray gene expression data. New York: Springer.

Lesk A. M. bioinformatics. Encyclopedia Britannica, Feb 16, 2023, https://www.britannica.com/science/bioinformatics. Accessed May 15, 2023.

Milgram, J. 2006. "One Against One" or "One Against All": Which One is Better for Handwriting Recognition with SVMs?. https://hal.archives-ouvertes.fr/inria-00103955/document access May 15, 2023.
Mohammed, M., Khan, MB., and Bashier, E. B. M., (2017). Machine Learning: Algorithms and Applications. CRC press. New York.
Morfouace M., Cheepala S., Jackson S., Fukuda Y., Patel Y. T., Fatima S., Kawauchi D,. Shelat A. A., Stewart C. F., Sorrentino B. P., Schuetz J. D., Roussel M. F., (2015), ABCG2 Transporter Expression Impacts Group 3 Medulloblastoma Response to Chemotherapy. *Cancer Res* 2015 Sep 15;75(18):3879–89. PMID: 26199091.
Paul A. Northcott, Andrey Korshunov, Hendrik Witt, Thomas Hielscher, Charles G. Eberhart, Stephen Mack, Eric Bouffet, Steven C. Clifford, Cynthia E. Hawkins, Pim French, James T. Rutka, Stefan Pfister, and Michael D. Taylor, (2011). Medulloblastoma comprises four distinct molecular variants, *Journal of Clinical Oncology*, 29(11), https://www.ncbi.nlm.nih.gov/pmc/articles/PMC4874239/pdf/zlj 1408.pdf. Access May 15, 2023.
Nugroho, A. S. 2003. Suport Vector Machines : Teori Aplikasinya dalam Bioinformatika ilmukomputer.com.
Perry J. S. (2017). What is big data? More than volume, velocity, and variety, https://developer.ibm.com/blogs/what-is-big-data-more-than-volume-velocity-and-variety/ access May 15, 2023.
Robinson G., Parker M., Kranenburg T. A., Lu C., Chen X., Ding L., Phoenix T. N., Hedlund E., Wei L., Zhu X., Chalhoub N., Baker S. J., Huether R., Kriwacki R., Curley N., Thiruvenkatam R., Wang J., Wu G., Rusch M., Hong X., Becksfort J, Gupta P., Ma J., Easton J., Vadodaria B., Onar-Thomas A., Lin T, Li S, Pounds S., Paugh S., Zhao D., Kawauchi D., Roussel M. F., Finkelstein D., Ellison D. W., Lau C. C., Bouffet E., Hassall T., Gururangan S., Cohn R., Fulton R. S., Fulton L. L., Dooling D. J., Ochoa K., Gajjar A., Mardis E. R., Wilson R. K., Downing J. R., Zhang J., Gilbertson R. J. Novel mutations target distinct subgroups of Medulloblastoma. *Nature* 2012 Aug 2;488(7409):43-8. PMID: 22722829.
Rossi A., Caracciolo V., Russo G., Reiss K., Giordano A. (2008). Medulloblastoma: from molecular pathology to therapy. *Clin Cancer Res* 14:971–976.
Upadhyay, A. K. (2014). Pediatric Medulloblastoma: Molecular biology, correlation with the histopathological and clinical outcome http://dspace.sctimst.ac.in/jspui/bitstream/123456789/2637/1/6307.pdf accessed pada 24 Oktober 2017.
Zhang, A. (2006). Advanced analysis of gene expression microarray data. Singapore: World Scientific Publishing.

Chapter 6

Prostate Cancer Biomarkers

Maxim N. Peshkov[1,*] and Igor V. Reshetov[2]

[1]Chair of Oncology and Plastic Surgery, Academy of Postgraduate Education, FGBU FSCC FMBA of Russia, Moscow, Russia
[2]Chair of Oncology, Radiotherapy and Reconstructive Surgery, I. M. Sechenov First MSMU MOH Russia, (Sechenovskiy University), Moscow, Russia

Abstract

PSA is the most widely used diagnostic and prognostic prostate cancer (PCa) biomarker. Since the "era of prostate-specific antigen (PSA)," we have seen an increase in unnecessary biopsies, ultimately leading to overtreatment of low-risk cancers.

Given the diagnostic limitations of the PSA test and its derivatives and the invasive nature of prostate biopsy, several serum and urine biomarkers have been developed.

This review provides a comprehensive overview of available biomarkers for detecting clinically significant prostate cancer: PHI, 4Kscore, PCA3, MiPS, SelectMDx, and ExosomeDX.

These tests focus on diagnosing clinically significant prostate cancer, trying to test and calibrate application algorithms in different populations.

There needs to be more evidence for the impact of magnetic resonance imaging (MRI) for early diagnosis and combination with these new markers and its possible role in disease screening, and not just in the early diagnosis process. In addition, only a few studies directly compare these tests with each other, and with PSA, so there needs to be more evidence to know which test has the best properties in each clinical

---

[*] Corresponding Author's Email: drpeshkov@gmail.com.

In: A Closer Look at Cancer Biomarkers
Editor: Arli Aditya Parikesit
ISBN: 979-8-89113-497-3
© 2024 Nova Science Publishers, Inc.

scenario. In the current scenario, prospective comparative studies in different populations are needed to evaluate their clinical usefulness in combination with MRI and fusion biopsy to elucidate the proper diagnostic role of these new biomarkers.

Modern molecular genetic testing improves clinically significant prostate cancer verification, reducing overtreatment and making treatment strategies more cost-effective. However, extensive prospective studies with head-to-head comparisons of available biomarkers are needed to fully evaluate the potential for incorporating biomarkers into routine clinical practice.

Keywords: prostate tumours, circulating extracellular DNA, microRNA, RNA marker, biomarker, metabolomics, multiplex analysis of urine markers

Introduction

Prostate cancer is the most common non-cutaneous malignancy in men. Traditionally, prostate-specific antigen (PSA) has been used for disease screening, while prostate biopsy is required for diagnosis. However, PSA specificity is only 20–45% (Kazutoshi and Nonomura 2018), resulting in many unnecessary prostate biopsies.

The limitations of screening tools, primarily serum prostate-specific antigen (PSA), have been widely proven.

Many low-risk prostate cancers are only suitable for surveillance, so there is an urgent need for minimally invasive prostate cancer biomarkers to accurately distinguish low-risk cancer from aggressive disease.

The negative predictive value of PSA is only 85%. Among patients screened for PSA 2.5 to 10 ng/mL (and abnormal FR), 75% have a negative biopsy (Bozeman et al. 2005).

Conversely, 10 to 35% of these patients are later diagnosed with prostate adenocarcinoma during repeat biopsies. The use of velocity (PSAv), PSA density (PSAd), age-related PSA, complex PSA (PSAc), and free/total PSA ratio brought only marginal diagnostic improvements. These limitations fuel debate about the relevance of mass screening for prostate cancer, which has been shown to reduce specific mortality by 20% but also highlights the risk of overdiagnosis and overtreatment (Schröder et al. 2009).

Urine biomarkers are attractive because prostate cancer cells are shed in urine, making screening minimally invasive. Urine biomarkers also evaluate the entire prostate, unlike a prostate biopsy, which is a small part of the cancer. Accurate urine biomarkers further minimize unnecessary prostate biopsies by pinpointing which prostate cancers require aggressive treatment.

The development of new PCa markers is urgently needed to improve the detection of the disease and the isolation of aggressive forms requiring treatment. Over the past ten years, the invasive approach of tissue examination and biopsy was abandoned, and much interest has focused on markers from biological fluids, particularly urine. These fluids represent a more accurate reflection of the polyclonal nature of prostate tumours than a random tissue sample. They contain both degradation products of benign and malignant cells and their protein secretion. Finally, affordable and minimally invasive urine collection makes these markers ideal candidates for mass screening. Thus, three groups of urinary markers can be distinguished: DNA, RNA, and protein markers.

Urine as a Potential Source for the Detection of Prostate Cancer Biomarkers

End of the previous paragraph. Body fluids potentially useful for screening for PCa include prostate secretions, semen, serum, and urine. In prostate cancer, metabolites and epithelial cells are released into body fluids, especially when the prostate is physically manipulated (massaged). This event presents an opportunity for noninvasive urine or prostate secretions detection. Urine, as a biomaterial, is readily available, noninvasive, and represents a promising source of biomarkers.

Blood and urine comprise two compartments, cellular and extracellular, each containing nucleic acids. Compartments can be roughly separated by a conventional centrifugation step into blood clot/cells, serum/plasma, urine supernatant and urinary sediment. In the case of cancer patients, nucleic acids released from cancer cells are usually found in serum/plasma or urine supernatant as extracellular nucleic acids, while tumour cells separated from cancer may occur in the cellular compartment in addition to blood or normal cells. Cells of the urogenital tract in the urine could be affected as well. This review summarizes recent aspects of urinary nucleic acid markers.

> supernatant - a liquid above a solid layer (sediment, sediment) after centrifugation or sedimentation (Firsov 2006).

The main advantages of urine tests are their noninvasive nature and the ability to monitor prostate cancer with heterogeneous foci. Nearly all urinary-specific prostate markers have recently been reviewed. For this reason, we will only focus here on a few promising markers that have been independently evaluated (particularly PCA3, fusion genes, TERT, AMACR, GSTP1, MMP9, and VEGF) and on the most recent markers (ANXA3 and sarcosine).

Emphasis is also placed on multiplex biomarker analysis and microarray-based fusion gene analysis. A combination of several urinary biomarkers may be helpful in men with persistently elevated serum prostate-specific antigen and a history of negative biopsy results. Emerging urine tests should help both in the early diagnosis of prostate cancer and in identifying aggressive tumours for radical treatment (Jamaspishvili et al. 2010).

DNA and RNA represent extracellular nucleic acids (CNAs) or circulating nucleic acids (from English, cell-free nucleic acids, cDNAs). Numerous studies in various scientific centres have shown that determining the level of cfDNA allows the diagnosis of various forms of the tumour process, assessing the degree of its severity or the risk of metastasis (Urbanova et al. 2010).

Origin and Presence of Nucleic Acids in Body Fluids

The presence of extracellular or circulating nucleic acids (ecNA) in the blood was discovered in 1948 by Mandel P., Metals P. (Mandel and Metals 1948). Later, cfNAs were found in plasma, blood serum, and urine. In the blood and urine of healthy individuals, cfNAs are found in free form and adsorbed on blood cells and epithelial cells (Tokareva et al. 2007).

Since the discovery of the presence of human extracellular or circulating nucleic acids (RNA) in blood and other biological fluids (liquor, lymph, urine, and others.), studies have been carried out not only on their biological role but also on the possibility of using them as diagnostic indicators for various pathological conditions. States of cfNK are considered potential diagnostic, prognostic, and predictive cancer biomarkers (Kondratova et al. 2013).

It has been established that the content of circulating nucleic acids changes in diabetes, myocardial infarction, systemic lupus erythematosus, rheumatoid arthritis, glomerulonephritis, hepatitis, and other pathological conditions (Tong and Lo 2006).

Abo-El-Eneen M.S. et al. showed that the concentration of cfDNA in the blood of patients with malignant neoplasms exceeded that of healthy individuals and patients with benign tumours (Abo-El-Eneen et al. 2013). After radiation therapy, the level of cfDNA decreased in patients with cancer of the lungs, ovaries, uterus, breast, and others., but the degree of decrease varied significantly. In patients who did not respond to anticancer therapy, the content of cfDNA in the blood serum remained at a high level or continued to increase. It was shown that patients with a high level of cfDNA after treatment had an unfavourable prognosis (Paci et al. 2009).

The cfDNA content in patients' blood after surgical treatment of tumours was analyzed. In patients without relapses after surgical treatment, the content of cfDNA decreased. In patients in whom the disease progressed, the level of cfDNA remained high (Szpechcinski et al. 2012).

Circulating nucleic acids are represented by both DNA and RNA. Numerous studies have been carried out in various research centres, and it has been shown that determining the level of cfDNA allows the diagnosis of various forms of the tumour process by assessing its severity or the risk of metastasis (Urbanova et al. 2010). RNAs circulating in the blood of healthy individuals are part of an open network of non-coding regulatory RNAs whose primary function is to mediate between DNA and proteins.

In a study by Hung E. C. W. et al., the presence of microRNAs belonging to the family of small non-coding regulatory RNAs in the blood of healthy individuals and patients with prostate cancer was shown. MicroRNA detection is of interest, and as technology continues to evolve, plasma (and urine) may replace tissue to diagnose prostate adenocarcinoma (Hung et al. 2009). To this end, the next step is to introduce ctDNA into everyday practice to realize liquid biopsy's full potential as a precision medicine diagnostic tool.

Genomic and mitochondrial DNA and RNA, including specific messenger ribonucleic acid (mRNA), small non-coding RNA molecules (miRNA), and long non-coding RNA molecules (lncRNA), are found as cell-free molecular components in urine samples from healthy individuals and cancer patients (Garcia-Olmo DC and Garcia-Olmo D 2013). A schematic overview of nucleic acids of interest released from cells and present as cfNA in blood or urine is shown in Figure 1.

The origin of cfNK in the blood and urine, both under normal and pathological conditions, remains open.

Today, three main processes can lead to the appearance of cfDNA in the blood: necrosis, apoptosis, and release from intact cells (Zaitsev and Skvortsov 2009).

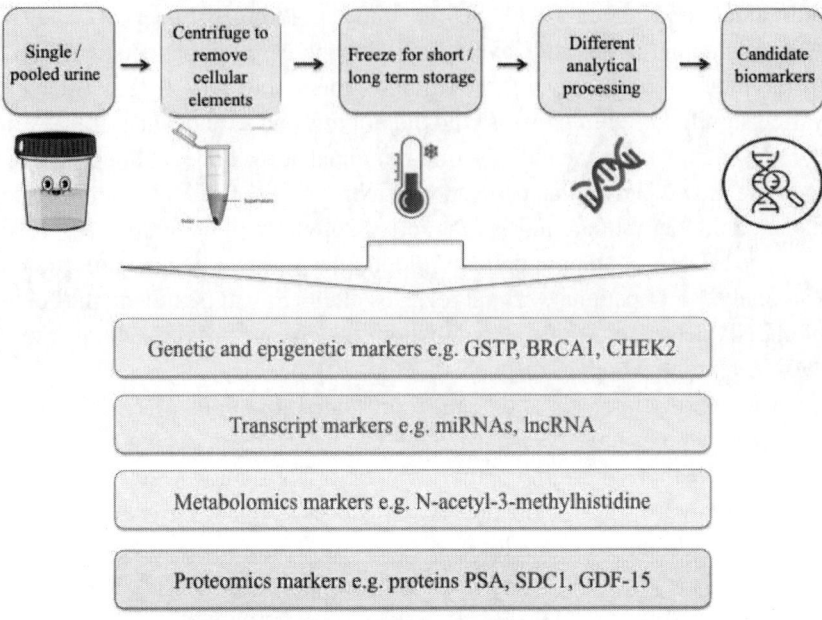

Figure 1. Preanalytical and analytical stages of the study of biomarkers in urine.

Necrosis may be responsible for the appearance of extracellular DNA in plasma and urine, although it is unlikely that necrotic cells provide much of the plasma DNA in healthy individuals.

Deligezer U. et al. (Deligezer et al. 2006) indicate the presence of fragmented nucleosomal DNA in the blood of patients with lymphoma and multiple myeloma. An increase in the level of nucleosomes that are released into the blood from dying cells under various pathological conditions has been reported in other studies (Holdenrieder and Stieber 2009).

Determination of nucleosomes in circulating blood has been proposed to be used for diagnosis, staging, and monitoring in cancer treatment (Deligezer et al. 2006).

In vivo and in vitro studies using Jurkat cell culture showed that the rate of NA release from apoptotic or necrotic cells changes significantly in the presence of macrophages, under the action of hormones and some chemicals, and also under conditions of inflammation (Pisetsky and Jiang 2006).

Ning Jiang et al. suggested that intense cell death induces macrophage apoptosis, which releases nuclear material from both engulfed but incompletely digested cells and the macrophages themselves. According to the authors, this explains the appearance of both cfDNA and nucleosomes in the bloodstream (Jiang et al. 2003).

In contrast to the partially understood cellular biogenetic pathways of various nucleic acids, they are described in detail in the corresponding review (Rykova et al. 2012). Tissue biomarkers based on nucleic acids that lead to changes in the processes of extracellular nucleic acids when they are translocated from cells, normal or malignant, into the systemic circulation are largely unknown (Rykova et al. 2012).

It has been suggested that several processes lead to changes in cfNAs in cancer patients (Figure 2) (Jung et al. 2010).

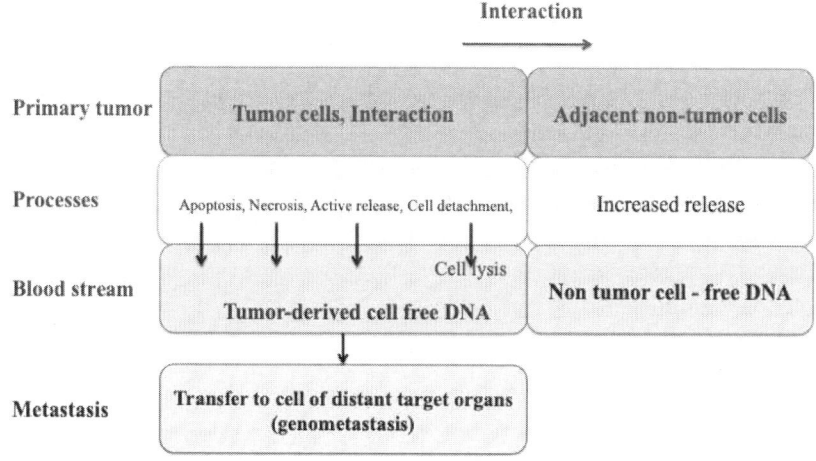

Figure 2. Formation of circulating cfNAs in cancer patients (adapted from Jung K. et al.).

These processes may differ for extracellular DNA (ecDNA) and extracellular RNA (ecRNA) since DNA in the blood occurs in free, naked form and the form of particles. At the same time, RNA is found mainly in the form of particles (Pisetsky and Ullal 2010).

These changes in body fluids (blood, urine) reflect a "disturbance of homeostasis" and serve as the basis for their potential use as biomarkers, which are defined as "a biological property of a person or animal, the measurement or identification of which in vitro is useful for prevention, diagnosis, prognosis," treatment and follow-up of diseases in humans or animals, as well as to understand their development" (Fuentes-Arderiu 2013).

In this regard, quantitative changes in total cfDNA, qualitative changes in cfDNA such as methylation, microsatellite, and mutational changes, as well as RNA changes with, for example, an increase or decrease in the occurrence of one or more mRNAs or microRNAs that are characteristic of tumours, are strongly influenced by methodological approaches. Aspects. Thus, the common points that prevent using these changes as biomarkers are critically discussed in the next section and discussed in more detail in the tumour-related sections.

DNA and Genomics of Prostate Cancer

Liquid biopsy opens up new possibilities for detecting, analyzing, and monitoring cancer in various bodily secretions, such as blood or urine, instead of a piece of cancerous tissue. It comprises various biological matrices such as circulating tumour cells (CTCs), cell-free nucleic acids, exosomes, or tumour "formed platelets." In addition to presenting a noninvasive or minimally invasive procedure, it should provide a better understanding of tumour heterogeneity and enable real-time tracking of cancer progression. Recent technological and molecular advances, greatly facilitated in many cases by the use of microfluidics, have allowed significant advances in our ability to purify and analyze the liquid components of a biopsy. In particular, significant developments in drop-based digital PCR and various optimizations of next-generation sequencing technologies are central to several validations of CTC-free DNA as a potent cancer biomarker.

The analysis of genetic changes in cancer currently occupies a central place in diagnosing and choosing treatment tactics for a cancer patient (Hofman and Popper 2016).

Moreover, intratumoral heterogeneity, especially spatial heterogeneity, can lead to unreliable biomarker detection results, especially when testing a single biopsy (Barranha et al. 2015). In addition, multiple tumour foci complicate the characterization of a patient's cancer. The availability of tumour specimens in long-term treatment patients may also be difficult, and in addition, testing archived tumour specimens may not be optimal due to tumour evolution. In addition, since serial monitoring of tumour progression and evolution in patients may be required, the reuse of tissue biopsy is only sometimes possible. Thus, there is an urgent need to use more accessible materials that involve noninvasive or minimally invasive procedures that allow systematic and real-time monitoring of molecular changes in cancer in a patient. Liquid biopsy represents the ideal procedure for such applications, as evidenced in large part by the impressive developments we have witnessed in recent years.

It is known that the circulating blood or urine of oncological patients contains various tumour-associated components, including tumour cells, non-tumour epithelial cells from the host organ, endothelial cells, and nucleic acids, either in a free state or in a complex. With the protein part (Ilie et al. 2014).

In patients with prostate cancer, adenocarcinoma DNA is present in the urine. The urine precipitations contain prostate cancer cells or fragmented cells containing cancer DNA.

Nucleic acids are normal urine constituents in healthy individuals and patients with tumours. They are found in

1. cell fraction of urine after centrifugation;
2. extracellularly in the supernatant as cell-free nucleic acids or contained in
3. extracellular vesicles (exosomes) (Ralla et al. 2014).

Cancer detection using DNA-based markers focuses on identifying (1) cfDNA content or (2) cancer-specific changes (Ellinger et al. 2011).

Although elevated cfDNA levels are an almost universal hallmark of cancer, cancer-specific DNA changes have been considered to improve diagnostic specificity. Tumor-specific changes include (1) genetic and (2) epigenetic modifications (Muller and Brenner 2006).

Genetic. The methylation status of the glutathione CG island GSTP1 was analyzed in tissue samples after prostatectomy, and the GSTP1 CG island was methylated in prostate cancer samples (Lee et al. 1997). In urine precipitations obtained after prostate massage, hypermethylation of the GSTP1 promoter was found in 2% of 45 patients and diagnosed with BPH in 72% of 40 patients with prostate cancer (Goessl et al. 2001). The sensitivity and specificity of prostate cancer detection were 73% and 98%, respectively. Several groups have reported the significance of GSTP1 promoter hypermethylation in urine precipitations for the detection of prostate cancer (Nakayama et al. 2004).

Prostate adenocarcinoma DNA is present in extracellular form in the urine. Extracellular DNA was isolated from urine without prostate manipulation in patients with CRPC, and AR amplification was found in half of the patients (five out of ten) with CRPC. TMPRSS2-ERG fusion, deletion of the PTEN gene, amplification of the NOTCH1 locus, and amplification of

MYCL have also been detected in cell-free urine DNA from patients with CRPC (Xia et al. 2016).

Normal apoptotic cells are known to produce highly fragmented DNA, while cancer cells produce longer DNA inside the nucleus.

Although less than 10% of cfDNA originates from tumour cells, (Ellinger et al. 2008) substantial evidence exists for higher levels of circulating cfDN K in patients with cancer, including men with PCa. Diagnosis of prostate cancer with a sensitivity of 80% and a specificity of 82%; others similarly correlated cfDNA with Gleason score, extraprostatic extension, and pathological stage (Bastian et al. 2008).

It is known that in solid tumours, including prostate cancer, 250 bp is often amplified. in 3 regions: c-Myc (8q24.21), HER2 (17q12.1), and BCAS1 (20q13.2) (Tabach et al. 2011).

The advantage of the proposed approach is that extracellular DNA, as previously shown (Casadio et al. 2012), can be easily detected in very small amounts of urine. In addition, unlike protein or RNA, it has good stability and is inexpensive and noninvasive, with results available in about two business days. In the future, it could be used as a standalone test or, due to its high specificity, help detect cases of false-positive PSA, especially in a subgroup of individuals with a grey area of PSA values, thereby reducing the number of unnecessary invasive diagnostic tests (for example, prostate biopsy).

Existing results suggest that urinary cell-free DNA integrity is a potentially good marker for early diagnosis of noninvasive prostate cancer, with an overall diagnostic accuracy of about 80% (Muller and Brenner 2006).

This preliminary finding paves the way for more extensive case series confirmatory studies.

Given the pronounced molecular and spatial intratumoral heterogeneity of PCa, multiplex genomic DNA profiling is a more effective methodological approach than the study of each biomarker separately.

RNA Markers in Prostate Cancer

MicroRNAs (miRNAs) are a group of conserved single-stranded small non-coding RNAs (18–25 nucleotides) that act post-transcriptionally to regulate protein expression. miRNAs make essential contributions to gene regulation, and their expression levels often change in many disease models. MicroRNAs comprise about 1% of the genome but target approximately 30% of genes (Singh and Campbell 2013).

Unlike other more prominent members of the RNA family, miRNAs are inherently resistant to RNase activity due to their small size and distinctive structure. They are also very stable in FFPE tissues and can be detected in serum and plasma (Gordanpour et al. 2012).

According to the literature, there are about 50 types of miRNAs that are involved in the development of cancer. The suppression or absence of miRNA expression is the most common sign in a malignant process. They are supposed to work as tumour suppressor genes. For example, miRNA-145 suppression is associated with many malignant neoplasms, including prostate cancer (Suh et al. 2011).

mRNA and metabolite profiles differ between patients with benign and malignant prostate diseases. Due to the high tissue tumour specificity, these molecules can act as full-fledged diagnostic and prognostic markers of prostate cancer. MicroRNAs are stable molecules easily detected in any biological material (plasma, urine, saliva) using real-time PCR.

Prostate Cancer Antigen PCA3

Prostate cancer antigen 3 (PCA3) is the most widely used urinary marker for prostate cancer. PCA3 was initially discovered as DD3 in 1999 by Bussemakers et al. They used differential display analysis to compare mRNA expression patterns in normal and malignant prostate tissues and identified DD3 cDNA that was highly overexpressed in 53 of 56 prostate cancer samples. For the quantitative determination of DD3, real-time PCR methods have been developed (Bussemakers et al. 1999). PCA3 and DD3 (PCA3) are found in urine precipitations after prostate massage. This test is based on a quantitative analysis of the RNA gene PCA3 (prostate cancer antigen 3, PCA3). This biomarker is a messenger RNA (mRNA), which in malignant cells is 60 times higher than in normal prostate cells but is present in minimal amounts in BPH cells (Fossati et al. 2015).

Based on European Association of Urology (EAU) recommendations, The PCA3 test is used in patients with a PSA level between 2.0 and 10.0 ng/mL before repeat prostate biopsy after a negative primary. However, additional studies and comparative analysis with other diagnostic markers are required. The US National Cancer Network recommends PCA3 as a secondary test to determine the need for a pancreatic biopsy (Carroll et al. 2016). The PCA3 test has been introduced into clinical practice in the Russian Federation, but the timing and indications for determining this test are not regulated.

Table 1. Commercialized urine-based biomarker tests for PCa

Test, Name	Company	Year	Biomarker	Material	Clinical Significance	Target patient	Technique
ExoDx Prostate (IntelliScore)	Exosome Diagnostics, Inc., Waltham, MA	2016	Exosomal RNA or expression of PCA3, TMPRSS2-ERG, SPDEF	Urine after DRE	Differential diagnosis of latent (less than 15.6 points) from aggressive (more than 15.6 points) cancer	Patient over 50 with PSA 4-10 ng/ml	Sequencing of RNA from extracellular vesicles
SelectMDx	MDxHealth, Irvine, CA	2016	Expression of DLX1, HOXC6, TDRD1	Urine after DRE	The test detects aggressive PCa (Gleason score ≥7)	Decision on primary biopsy in patients with PSA 4-10 ng/mL	RT-PCR
Michigan Prostate Score	The University of Michigan Comprehensive Cancer Center, USA	2013	Expression of PSA, T2MPRSS:ER, PCA3	Urine after DRE	Cancer-specific test (AUC 0.85) for verification of aggressive prostate cancer (Gleason ≥7) A score of 0 to 100 reflects the likelihood of finding cancer on a biopsy.	Verification of clinically significant prostate cancer (Gleason ≥7)	PSA in blood, PCA3 (mRNA) in urine and TMPRSS2:ERG (mRNA) in urine
Prostarix risk score	Metabolon, Durham, NC, USA	2013	Metabolites: sarcosine, glycine, alanine and glutamate.	Urine after DRE	Algorithm for assessing (from 0 to 100) the probability of cancer based on the results of prostate biopsy.	Increases the cancer specificity of the study in patients with PSA 4-10 ng/ml and a negative DRE	Investigation of urine sediment after DR by mass spectrometry and liquid chromatography
PTEN/TMPRSS2:ERG	Metamark, Waltham, MA, USA	2010	Fusion gene TMPRSS2:ERG and the tumor suppressor gene PTEN	Urine after DRE	Used in Gleason primary biopsy positive patients (3+3 or 3+4), with atypical/HGPIN	High-Risk Tumor Prediction	The presence of TMPRSS2:ERG and/or the absence of PTEN indicates a more aggressive cancer
PROGENSA PCA3	Gen-Probe Inc., San Diego, CA, USA	2012	ncRNA of PCA3 gene	Urine after DRE	Quantitative determination of PCA3 gene ncRNA in urine in patients with negative primary biopsy results	Update of tumor progression for repeat biopsy	TRF RT-PCR (The APTIMA® PCA3)

Prostate cancer antigen 3 (PCA3) is a validated urine biomarker that is used in several commercially available tests, such as PROGENSA PCA3, Michigan Prostate Score (MiPS), and ExoDx Prostate (IntelliScore). Table 1 shows urinary commercial RNA tests. PCA3 levels are beneficial for early detection of prostate cancer. Tosoian J.J. et al. showed that the PCA3 score obtained during AS was higher in men who underwent Gleason reclassification (GS), suggesting that PCA3 provides additional prognostic information in the setting of AS (Tosoian et al. 2010).

A PCA3-based nomogram for predicting prostate and high-grade prostate cancer at the initial biopsy has also been developed using information on age, serum PSA level, prostate volume, and PCA3 level (Greene et al. 2016).

Including PCA3 in the nomogram increased the accuracy of prostate cancer detection by 4.5–7.1%. PCA3 scores obtained at first biopsy and during active follow-up were significantly higher in patients with Gleason reclassification than in patients without this reclassification, but the longitudinal change in PCA3 score during active follow-up did not differ depending on Gleason score status (Tosoian et al. 2017).

Proteomic and Metabolic Markers of Prostate Cancer

Metabolic analysis is a modern biochemical methodological approach that allows analyzing the entire metabolic profile of a biological system. Because neoplastic cells have a unique metabolic phenotype associated with cancer development and progression, identifying dysfunctional metabolic pathways through metabolomics can be used to discover cancer biomarkers and therapeutic targets.

This section discusses urine metabolomics to detect changes in the metabolic phenotype of PCa and, thus, discover new biomarkers for diagnosing PCa. Promising results using metabolomics have been obtained for PCa, with sarcosine being one of the most promising biomarkers identified to date. However, using sarcosine as a biomarker for PCa in the clinic remains controversial in the scientific community. In addition to sarcosine, other metabolites are biomarkers for PCa, but they still need to be clinically tested. Despite the lack of metabolomic biomarkers that have reached clinical practice, metabolomics has proven to be a powerful tool for discovering new biomarkers for detecting PCa.

Systems biology applied in cancer research includes "omics" tools, including genomics, transcriptomics, proteomics, and metabolomics, which complement each other and can simultaneously measure changes in several entities (genes, transcripts, proteins or metabolites, respectively)—providing an overview of various physiological or pathological conditions (Halama 2014).

Metabolomics can provide insight into the physiological status of a biological system, and therefore, changes in "normal" metabolism may indicate disease. These changes in the "normal" metabolome may provide new diagnostic markers for disease detection and prognosis and for monitoring response to therapeutic interventions (Ramautar et al. 2013).

The term metabolomics includes the evaluation of all endogenous metabolites produced by the body, including small molecular weight intermediates and end products of biochemical reactions in the cell (approximately ≤ 1500 Da), as well as exogenous metabolites such as drugs, waste products of the body, and nutrition. Instead of the genes and proteins involved in these biological processes, the metabolites produced are indicators of what is going on in the cell's metabolism under physiological or pathophysiological conditions. Thus, metabolites can be altered in cancer-related diseases (Monteiro et al. 2013).

Because tumour cells have a unique metabolic phenotype associated with cancer development and progression, identifying dysfunctional metabolic pathways by metabolomics can be used to identify cancer biomarkers and discover therapeutic targets (Monteiro et al. 2014).

Metabolomic Studies in PCa Model Systems and Biological Fluids

Using urine as a sample for metabolomic studies has many advantages over serum: urine is easier to obtain and process, requires less sample preparation, has a higher amount of metabolites, and has a lower protein content (Zhang et al. 2013).

Metabolites Markers in Prostate Cancer

Several urinary metabolites have been analyzed as markers to improve the diagnosis and detection of PCa progression, including but not limited to alanine, aspartate, and glutamate (Lee et al. 2020). In addition, several studies have found decreased levels of glycine, glutamine, tyrosine, and citrate and elevated levels of valine, taurine, and leucine in the urine of PCa patients (Lima et al. 2021).

Prostarix Risk Assessment

It is a biomarker test that determines the concentration of 4 metabolites (sarcosine, glycine, alanine, and glutamate) in the urine to obtain a risk score from 0 to 100 that predicts the chances of detecting PCa on prostate biopsy (Malik et al. 2019).

One of the most recent PCa markers, annexin A3 (ANXA3), belongs to a family of calcium- and phospholipid-binding proteins that are involved in cell differentiation and migration, immunomodulation, bone formation, and mineralization during PCa metastasis. The presence of ANXA3 in urinary exosomes and protostomes may be responsible for its remarkable stability in urine.30 ANXA3 has been quantified by Western blotting in urine samples from patients with negative digital rectal examination (DRE) results and low total PSA (2–10 ng/mL), who represent a clinically significant group facing the biopsy dilemma (Schostak et al. 2009).

The combined PSA and urine ANXA3 values produced the best results in the area under the ROC curve of 0.82 for the total PSA range of 2-6 ng/mL, 0.83 for the total PSA range of 4-10 ng/mL, and 0.81 in all patients. ANXA3 has an inverse relationship with cancer; hence, its specificity was much better than that of PSA. It has been reported that the pattern of ANXA3 staining in prostate tissue correlates with the Gleason score and allows differentiation to cite lower and higher prostatic intraepithelial neoplasia (PIN) malignancies at various stages of prostate cancer.

Multiplex Analysis of Urine Markers and Further Directions

The multiplex or combined model of urine biomarker analysis has several advantages in prostate cancer detection. Most importantly, it does not ignore PCa heterogeneity and can detect prostate cancer more accurately than single marker tests (Schmidt et al. 2006).

Combining urine biomarkers may increase clinical value and provide a more reliable assessment of the heterogeneity inherent in prostate cancer.

PCA3 and TMPRSS2-ERG fusion testing increases sensitivity to 73 per cent (from 65 per cent) while maintaining high specificity for TMPRSS2-ERG8 fusion alone. This dual approach has been shown to reduce unnecessary prostate biopsies by up to 42 per cent (Kazutoshi and Nonomura 2018).

Laxman et al. (Laxman et al. 2008) reported that a multiplex panel of urinary transcripts outperformed only serum PCA3 and PSA transcripts in detecting PCa. Expression of seven putative prostate cancer biomarkers (PCA3, PSA, GOLPH2, SPINK1, AMACR, TMPRSS2/ERG, TFF3) was measured by qRT-PCR in urine samples. Inhibitor, Kasal type 1), PCA3 transcript expression, and TMPRSS2/ERG fusion status were significant predictors of CaP (66% sensitivity and 76% specificity). Urinary transcripts in a patient sample with serum PSA X3 ng/mL and abnormal DRE (Hessels et al. 2007). The sensitivity for detecting the fusion of TMPRSS2/ERG and PCA3 transcripts in urine was 37% and 62%, respectively, and the sensitivity of markers increased to 73%.

Conclusion

Urine is readily available and can be used to detect shedding cancer cells or secreted products. The main advantages of urine-based tests are their noninvasive nature and the ability to monitor prostate cancer with heterogeneous foci. Urinary bil markers allow monitoring of prostate cancer with heterogeneous foci and provide a noninvasive alternative to multiple biopsies. Even if a urinalysis cannot detect a cancer that does not shed tumour cells into the urine, it still deserves significant attention.

Advanced technologies such as NGS and machine learning have created a wide range of urine biomarkers for prostate cancer. Multiplex panels currently under development combine classes of biomarkers such as proteins and nucleic acids and use a more comprehensive range of known mutational abnormalities and available biomarkers. Challenges remain to validate and normalize the numerous available biomarkers while improving sensitivity and specificity.

Combining several urinary biomarkers may be essential in men with persistently elevated serum PSA levels and a history of negative biopsy results. New biomarkers (ANXA3, sarcosine, gene fusions, and PCA3) should help diagnose early prostate cancer by detecting aggressive tumour forms for radical treatment and avoiding unnecessary biopsies. The routine use of urine biomarkers in prostate cancer will increase the male population's duration and quality of life.

Acknowledgment

The authors thank the Academy of Postgraduate Education staff under FSCC of FMBA of RUSSIA, Moscow, and Sechenovskiy University, Moscow, for their heartfelt support in writing this manuscript.

All authors declare that they have no competing interests and have approved this manuscript's final version.

References

Barranha R., Costa J. L., Carneiro F., Machado J. C. 2015. Genetic heterogeneity in colorectal cancer and its clinical implications. *Acta Med Port.* 28(3):370–5. https://doi.org/10.20344/amp.5398.

Bastian P. J., Palapattu G. S., Yegnasubramanian S., Rogers C. G., Lin X., Mangold L. A., Trock B., Eisenberger M. A., Partin A. W., Nelson W. G. (2008). CpG island hypermethylation profile in the serum of men with clinically localized and hormone-refractory metastatic prostate cancer. *J Urol.* 179(2):529–34. https://doi.org/10.1016/j.juro.2007.09.038.

Bozeman C. B., Carver B. S., Caldito G., Venable D. D., Eastham J. A. 2005. Prostate cancer in patients with an abnormal digital rectal examination and serum prostate-specific antigen less than 4.0 ng/mL. *Urology.* 66:803-73. https://doi.org/10.1016/j.urology.2005.04.058.

Bussemakers M. J., van Bokhoven A., Verhaegh G. W., Smit F. P., Karthaus H. F., Schalken J. A., Debruyne F. M., Ru N., Isaacs W. B. 1999. DD3: a new prostate-specific gene, highly overexpressed in prostate cancer. *Cancer Res.* 59:5975–9.

Casadio V., Calistri D., Tebaldi M., Bravaccini S., Gunelli R., Martorana G., Bertaccini A., Serra L., Scarpi E., Amadori D., Silvestrini R., Zoli W. 2012. Urine Cell-Free DNA integrity as a marker for early bladder cancer diagnosis: preliminary data. *Urologic Oncology.* 31(8):1744-50. https://doi.org/10.1016/j.urolonc.2012.07.013.

Deligezer U., Erten N., Akisik E. E., Dalay N. 2006. Circulating fragmented nucleosomal DNA and caspase-3 mRNA in patients with lymphoma and myeloma. *Exp Mol Pathol.* 80(1):72-6. https://doi.org/10.1016/j.yexmp.2005.05.001.

Ellinger J., Haan K., Heukamp L. C., Kahl P., Büttner R., Müller S. C., von Ruecker A., Bastian P. J. 2008. CpG island hypermethylation in cell-free serum DNA identifies patients with localized prostate cancer. *Prostate.* 68(1):42–9. https://doi.org/10.1002/pros.20651.

Ellinger J., Muller S. C., Stadler T. C. Jung A., von Ruecker A., Bastian P. J. 2011. The role of cell-free circulating DNA in the diagnosis and prognosis of prostate cancer. *Urol Oncol.* 29(2):124–9. https://doi.org/10.1016/j.urolonc.2009.05.010.

Firsov N. N. (2006). *Microbiology: a dictionary of terms.* M: Bustard, (in Russian).

Fossati N., Buffi N. M., Haese A., Stephan C., Larcher A., McNicholas T., de la Taille A., Freschi M., Lughezzani G., Abrate A., Bini V., Palou Redorta J., Graefen M., Guazzoni G., Lazzeri M. 2015. Preoperative Prostate-specific Antigen Isoform p2PSA and Its Derivatives, %p2PSA and Prostate Health Index, Predict Pathologic Outcomes in Patients Undergoing Radical Prostatectomy for Prostate Cancer: Results from a Multicentric European Prospective Study. *Eur Urol.* 68(1):132–138. https://doi.org/10.1016/j.eururo.2014.07.034.

Fuentes-Arderiu X. 2013. What is a biomarker? It is time for a renewed definition. *Clin Chem Lab Med.* 51:1689–90. https://doi.org/10.1515/cclm-2013-0240.

Fujita, Kazutoshi and Norio Nonomura. 2018. Urinary biomarkers of prostate cancer. *International Journal of Urology.* 25.9:770–79. https://doi.org/10.1111/iju.13734.

Garcia-Olmo D. C., Garcia-Olmo D. 2013. Biological role of cell-free nucleic acids in cancer: the theory of genometastasis. *Crit Rev Oncol.* 18:153–61. https://doi.org/10.1615/critrevoncog.v18.i1-2.90.

Goessl C., MЄuller M., Heicappell R., Krause H., Straub B., Schrader M., Miller K. (2001). DNA-based detection of prostate cancer in urine after prostatic massage. *Urology.* 58:335–8. https://doi.org/10.1016/s0090-4295(01)01268-7.

Gordanpour A., Nam R., Seth A. (2012). MicroRNAs in prostate cancer: from biomarkers to molecularly-based therapeutics. *Prostate Cancer Prostatic Dis.* 2012:1–6. https://doi.org/10.1038/pcan.2012.3.

Greene D. J., Elshafei A., Nyame Y. A. Kara O., Malkoc E., Gao T., Jones J. S. 2016. External validation of a PCA-3-based nomogram for predicting prostate cancer and high-grade cancer on initial prostate biopsy. *Prostate.* 76:1019–23. https://doi.org/10.1002/pros.23197.

Halama A. (2014). Metabolomics in cell culture - a strategy to study crucial metabolic pathways in cancer development and the response to treatment. *Arch Biochem Biophys.* 564:100–109. https://doi.org/10.1016/j.abb.2014.09.002.

Hessels D., Smit F. P., Verhaegh G. W., Witjes J. A., Cornel E. B., Schalken J. A. 2007. Detection of TMPRSS2-ERG fusion transcripts and prostate cancer antigen 3 in urinary sediments may improve diagnosis of prostate cancer. *Clin Cancer Res.* 13:5103–5108. https://doi.org/10.1158/1078-0432.CCR-07-0700.

Hofman P., Popper H. H. 2016. Pathologists and liquid biopsies: to be or not to be? *Virchows Arch.* 469(6):601-609. https://doi.org/10.1007/s00428-016-2004-z.

Holdenrieder S., Stieber P. 2006. Clinical use of circulating nucleosomes. 2009. *Crit Rev Clin Lab Sci.* 46(1):1-24. https://doi.org/10.1080/10408360802485875.

Hung E. C. W., Chiu R. W. K., Lo Y. M. D. 2009. Detection of circulating fetal nucleic acids: a review of methods and applications. *J Clin Pathol.* 62:308–313. https://doi.org/10.1136/jcp.2007.048470.

Ilie M., Long E., Hofman V., Selva E., Bonnetaud C., Boyer J., Vénissac N., Sanfiorenzo C., Ferrua B., Marquette C. H., Mouroux J., Hofman P. 2014. Clinical value of circulating endothelial cells and soluble CD146 levels in patients undergoing surgery for non-small cell lung cancer. *Br J Cancer.* 110:1236–1243. https://doi.org/10.1038/bjc.2014.11.

Jamaspishvili T., Kral M., Khomeriki I., Student V., Kolar Z., Bouchal J.. (2010). Urine markers in monitoring for prostate cancer. *Prostate Cancer Prostatic Dis* 13(1):12–9. https://doi.org/10.1038/pcan.2009.31.

Jiang N., Reich C. F., Pisetsky D. S. 2003. Role of macrophages in the generation of circulating blood nucleosomes from dead and dying cells. *Blood.* 102 (6):2243–2250. https://doi.org/10.1182/blood-2002-10-3312.

Jung K., Fleischhacker M., Rabien A. 2010. Cell-free DNA in the blood as a solid tumor biomarker – a critical appraisal of the literature. *Clin Chim Acta.* 411:1611–24. https://doi.org/10.1016/j.cca.2010.07.032.

Kondratova V. N., Botezatu I. V., Shelepov V. P., Liechtenstein A. V. (2013). Extracellular nucleic acids as tumor growth markers. Russian biotherapeutic journal. No. 3. Vol. 12. p. 3-10. (in Russian).

Laxman B., Morris D. S., Yu J., Siddiqui J., Cao J., Mehra R., Lonigro R. J., Tsodikov A., Wei J. T., Tomlins S. A., Chinnaiyan A. M. (2008). A first-generation multiplex biomarker analysis of urine for the early detection of prostate cancer. *Cancer Res.* 68:645–649. https://doi.org/10.1158/0008-5472.CAN-07-3224.

Lee W. H., Isaacs W. B., Bova G. S., Nelson W. G. (1997). CG island methylation changes near the GSTP1 gene in prostatic carcinoma cells detected using the polymerase chain reaction: a new prostate cancer biomarker. *Cancer Epidemiol. Biomarkers Pre.* 6:443–50.

Lee B., Mahmud I., Marchica J., Derezinski P., Qi F., Wang F. Integrated RNA and metabolite profiling of urine liquid biopsies for prostate cancer biomarker discovery. *Sci Rep.* 2020;10(1):3716. https://doi.org/10.1038/s41598-020-60616-z.

Lima A. R., Pinto J., Amaro F., Bastos M. L., Carvalho M., Guedes de Pinho P. 2021. Advances and perspectives in prostate cancer biomarker discovery in the last 5 years through tissue and urine metabolomics. *Metabolites.* 11(3):181. https://doi.org/10.3390/metabo11030181.

Malik A., Srinivasan S., Batra J. 2019. A new era of prostate cancer precision medicine. *Front Oncol.* 9:1263. https://doi.org/10.3389/fonc.2019.01263.

Mandel P., Metais P. 1948. Les acides nucléiques du plasma sanguin chez l'homme [Nuclear Acids In Human Blood Plasma]. *C R Seances Soc Biol Fil.* 142(3-4):241-3. French. PMID: 18875018.

Monteiro M. S., Carvalho M., Bastos M. L., Guedes de Pinho P. 2013. Metabolomics analysis for biomarker discovery: advances and challenges. *Curr Med* Chem. 20:257–271. https://doi.org/10.2174/092986713804806621.

Monteiro M., Carvalho M., Henrique R., Jerónimo C., Moreira N., de Lourdes Bastos M., de Pinho P. G. 2014. Analysis of volatile human urinary metabolome by solid-phase microextraction in combination with gas chromatography–mass spectrometry for biomarker discovery: application in a pilot study to discriminate patients with renal cell carcinoma. *Eur J Cancer.* 50:1993–2002. https://doi.org/10.1016/j.ejca.2014.04.011.

Moses K. A., Sprenkle P. C., Bahler C. 2023. Journal of the National Comprehensive Cancer Network: *JNCCN*. Vol. 21, Issue 3, pages 236 – 246. https://doi.org/10.6004/jnccn.2023.0014.

Muller H., Brenner H. 2006. Urine markers as possible tools for prostate cancer screening: review of performance characteristics and practically. *Clin Chem.* 52(4):562–73. https://doi.org/10.1373/clinchem.2005.062919.

Nakayama M., Gonzalgo M. L., Yegnasubramanian S. 2004. GSTP1 CpG island hypermethylation as a molecular biomarker for prostate cancer. *J. Cell. Biochem.* 91:540–52. https://doi.org/10.1002/jcb.10740.

Paci M., Maramotti S., Bellesia E., Formisano D., Albertazzi L., Ricchetti T., Ferrari G., Annessi V., Lasagni D., Carbonelli C., De Franco S., Brini M., Sgarbi G., Lodi R. 2009. Circulating plasma DNA as diagnostic biomarker in non-small cell lung cancer. *Lung Cancer.* 64(1):92-7. https://doi.org/10.1016/j.lungcan.2008.07.012.

Pisetsky D. S., Jiang N. (2006). The Generation of Extracellular DNA in SLE: the Role of Death and Sex. *Scand J Immunol.* 64(3):200–4. https://doi.org/10.1111/j.1365-3083.2006.01822.x.

Pisetsky D. S., Ullal A. J. 2010. The blood nucleosome in the pathogenesis of SLE. *Autoimmun Rev.* 10:35–7. https://doi.org/10.1016/j.autrev.2010.07.007.

Ralla B., Stephan C., Meller S., Dietrich D., Kristiansen G., Jung K. 2014. Nucleic acid-based biomarkers in body fluids of patients with urologic malignancies. *Critical reviews in clinical laboratory sciences.* 51(4):200–231. https://doi.org/10.3109/10408363.2014.914888.

Ramautar R., Berger R., van der Greef J., Hankemeier T. 2013. Human metabolomics: strategies to understand biology. *Curr Opin Chem Biol.* 17:841–846. https://doi.org/10.1016/j.cbpa.2013.06.015.

Rykova E. Y., Morozkin E. S., Ponomaryova A. A., Loseva E. M., Zaporozhchenko I. A., Cherdyntseva N. V., Vlassov V. V., Laktionov P. P. 2012. Cell-free and cell-bound circulating nucleic acid complexes: mechanisms of generation, concentration, and content. *Expert Opin Biol Ther.* 12:S141–53. https://doi.org/10.1517/14712598.2012.673577.

Schmidt U., Fuessel S., Koch R., Baretton G. B., Lohse A., Tomasetti S., Unversucht S., Froehner M., Wirth M. P., Meye A. 2006. Quantitative multi-gene expression profiling of primary prostate cancer. *Prostate.* 66:1521–1534. https://doi.org/10.1002/pros.20490.

Schostak M, Schwall G. P., Poznanovic S., Groebe K., Müller M., Messinger D., Miller K., Krause H., Pelzer A., Horninger W., Klocker H., Hennenlotter J., Feyerabend S., Stenzl A, Schrattenholz A. 2009. Annexin A3 in urine: a highly specific noninvasive marker for prostate cancer early detection. *J Urol.* 181:343–353. https://doi.org/10.1016/j.juro.2008.08.119.

Schröder F. H., Hugosson J., Roobol M. J. ERSPC. 2009. Screening and prostate-cancer mortality in a randomized European study. *N Engl J Med.* 360:1320—8. https://doi.org/10.1056/NEJMoa0810084.

Singh P. K., Campbell M. J. (2013). The interactions of microRNA and epigenetic modifications in prostate cancer. *Cancers.* 5:998–1019. https://doi.org/10.3390/cancers5030998.

Suh S. O., Chen Y., Zaman M. S., Hirata H., Yamamura S., Shahryari V., Liu J., Tabatabai Z. L., Kakar S., Deng G., Tanaka Y., Dahiya R. 2011. MicroRNA-145 is regulated by DNA methylation and p53 gene mutation in prostate cancer. *Carcinogenesis.* 32(5):772–778. https://doi.org/10.1093/carcin/bgr036.

Szpechcinski A., Chorostowska-Wynimko J., Kupis W., Maszkowska-Kopij K., Dancewicz M., Kowalewski J., Orlowski T. 2012. Quantitative analysis of free circulating DNA in plasma of patients with resectable NSCLC. *Expert Opin. Biol. Ther.* 12 Suppl 1:S3-9. https://doi.org/10.1517/14712598.2012.668519.

Tabach Y., Sakin I. K., Buganim Y., Solomon H., Goldfinger N., Hovland R., Ke X. S., Oyan A. M., Kalland K. H., Rotter V., Domany E. 2011. Amplification of the 20q chromosomal arm occurs early in tumorigenic transformation and may initiate cancer. *PLoS ONE.* 6(1)e14632. https://doi.org/10.1371/journal.pone.0014632.

Tamkovich S. N., Laktionov P. P., Bryzgunova O. E., The level of extracellular nucleic acids associated with the surface of blood cells in the diagnosis of breast cancer. *Mol. Medicine.* - 2005. - No 2. - S. 46–50. (in Russian).

Tong Y. K., Lo Y. M. (2006). Diagnostic developments involving cell-free (circulating) nucleic acids. *Clin Chim Acta.* 363(1-2):187-96. https://doi.org/10.1016/j.cccn.2005.05.048.

Tosoian J. J., Loeb S., Kettermann A., Landis P., Elliot D. J., Epstein J. I., Partin A. W., Carter H. B., Sokoll L. J. 2010. Accuracy of PCA3 measurement in predicting short-term biopsy progression in an active surveillance program. *J Urol.* 183(2):534–8. https://doi.org/10.1016/j.juro.2009.10.003.

Tosoian J. J., Patel H. D., Mamawala M., Landis P., Wolf S., Elliott D. J., Epstein J. I., Carter H. B., Ross A. E., Sokoll L. J., Pavlovich C. P. 2017. Longitudinal assessment of urinary PCA3 for predicting prostate cancer grade reclassification in favorable-risk men during active surveillance. *Prostate Cancer Prostatic Dis.* 20:339–42. https://doi.org/10.1038/pcan.2017.16.

Urbanova, M., Plzak, J., Strnad, H., Betka J. 2010. Circulating nucleic acids as a new diagnostic tool. *Cell Mol Biol Lett.* 15, 242–259. https://doi.org/10.2478/s11658-010-0004-6.

Xia Y., Huang C.-C., Dittmar R., Du M., Wang Y., Liu H., Shenoy N., Wang L., Kohli M. 2016. Copy number variations in urine cell free DNA as biomarkers in advanced prostate cancer. *Oncotarget.* 7:35818–31. https://doi.org/10.18632/oncotarget.9027.

Zaher E. R., Anwar M. M., Kohail H. M. A., El-Zoghby S. M., Abo-El-Eneen M. S. 2013. Cell-free DNA concentration and integrity as a screening tool for cancer. *Indian Journal of Cancer.* 50(3):175-83. https://doi.org/10.4103/0019-509X.118721.

Zaitsev V. G., Skvortsov V. V. 2009. Prospects for the determination of DNA in serum or plasma for the diagnosis and monitoring of cancer. *Oncology.* 13;864. - S. 864-866. (in Russian).

Zhang T., Watson D. G., Wang L., Abbas M., Murdoch L., Bashford L., Ahmad I., Lam N. Y., Ng A. C., Leung H. Y. (2013). Application of holistic liquid chromatography–high-resolution mass spectrometry-based urinary metabolomics for prostate cancer detection and biomarker discovery. *PLoS One.* 8:e65880. https://doi.org/10.1371/journal.pone.0065880.

Chapter 7

Tissue Markers of Prostate Cancer (Review)

Maxim N. Peshkov[1,2,*]
and Igor V. Reshetov[1,2,†]

[1]Academy of Postgraduate Education under FSCC of FMBA of RUSSIA, Moscow, Russia
[2]I. M. Sechenov First MSMU MOH Russia (Sechenovskiy University), Moscow, Russia

Abstract

Prostate cancer is the most prevalent type of tumour in males. The commonly used blood test for prostate-specific antigen (PSA) assesses the efficiency of early disease detection. Overdiagnosis frequently leads to excessive or unjustified treatment. Clinical outcomes in patients with identical clinical and histological characteristics are difficult to predict. Prostate adenocarcinoma might be asymptomatic in the early stages. A prostate puncture biopsy and histological testing results remain the gold standard for diagnosis, prognosis, and treatment strategies. The efficiency of early detection determines cancer-specific survival and treatment results.

We can better identify the tumour process thanks to the advancement of molecular genetic technologies. PTEN/TMPRSS2:ERG, ConfirmMDx®, Prolaris®, Oncoytype DX®, Decipher®, and Promark® are only a few of the diagnostic and prognostic biomarkers that have been discovered for tumour verification in PCa. These test systems have aided tumour detection, prognosis, and clinical decision-making. The review focuses on commercially accessible prostate cancer tissue biomarkers. These markers are utilized for active patient follow-up, identifying

---

[*] Corresponding Author's Email: drpeshkov@gmail.com.
[†] Corresponding Author's Email: reshetoviv@mail.ru.

In: A Closer Look at Cancer Biomarkers
Editor: Arli Aditya Parikesit
ISBN: 979-8-89113-497-3
© 2024 Nova Science Publishers, Inc.

clinically significant illness, and deciding whether to employ salvage or adjuvant radiation following prostatectomy.

The primary goal of this study is to present an overview of current tissue markers utilized for prostate cancer (PC) diagnosis, prognosis, and prevention, as well as to explore their analytical capabilities.

Keywords: prostate cancer, molecular genetic markers, tissue biomarker, risk prediction, Prolaris®, ConfirmMDx®, Oncotype Dx®, Decipher®, Promark®

1.0. Introduction

Prostate cancer is the world's most significant cause of morbidity and mortality. It is the fifth and second most prevalent cause of death from malignant neoplasms in men [1]. Clinicians have employed biopsy to identify many disorders for thousands of years [2]. Histological examination remains the gold standard for diagnosing and staging prostate cancer [3].

Biopsy in cancer patients enables histological evaluation of the disease and, more recently, details of the tumour's genetic profile, which can predict the course of the disease and response to therapy. As the technologies for analyzing biopsies get more sophisticated, we are becoming more conscious of the limitations of looking at a single tumour image. Gerlinger et al. [4] demonstrated that sections collected from different regions of the primary tumour and its metastases show significant intertumoral and intratumoral development, emphasizing the bias of a single biopsy. This tumour heterogeneity highlights the challenge of deciding on a therapeutic course of action based on a single biopsy, which must most likely account for the complexity of the tumour's genomic landscape.

The Gleason score in diagnostic biopsy remains the most reliable tool for predicting prostate cancer. Patients are classed as low, moderate, or high when the Gleason score is combined with traditional clinical criteria such as serum PSA levels and clinical stage. Group at risk [5].

1.1. Prostate Cancer Heterogeneity and Biomarkers

Prostate cancer is distinguished by significant intratumoral heterogeneity and multifocal development. There are clear limitations in the use of biopsies for biomarker assessment. In 80% of original cases identified with a rise in blood PSA, multifocal development of heterogeneous prostate cancer foci is seen [6].

Most of the time, the prominent (index) lesion with the most significant volume and the highest Gleason score can be recognized. Other tumour foci are significantly smaller and have a lower Gleason score. Today, it has been demonstrated that the source of metastasis, rather than smaller tumour foci, is the primary focus of prostate cancer [7].

In addition to intertumoral heterogeneity, intratumoral heterogeneity often manifests morphologically, as more than one Gleason growth pattern may present in a single prostate cancer site (e.g., pattern three and pattern 4 in Gleason prostate cancer). With this variant of inter- and intra-tumoral heterogeneity, puncture biopsy of the prostate and histological examination can provide the following four scenarios (Figure 1):

1. Option 1 (3+3) 6 points on the Gleason scale (low risk);
2. Option 2 (3+4) 7 points on the Gleason scale (intermediate risk);
3. Option 3 (4+3) 7 points on the Gleason scale (intermediate risk);
4. Option 3 (4+4): 8 points on the Gleason scale (high risk).

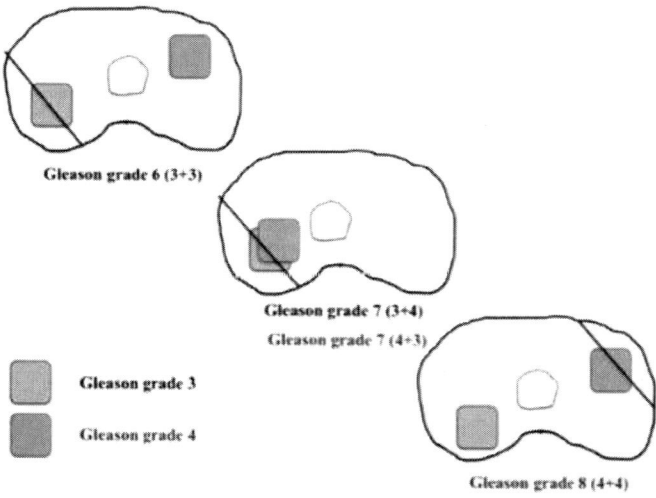

Figure 1. Sampling bias in puncture biopsy of the prostate.

In three scenarios, all needle biopsy rods of the prostate, as shown in the figures, will have an adenocarcinoma of 6 (3+3) on the Gleason score. It would be a correct Gleason estimate in Scenario I but an underestimate of Gleason's actual estimate in Scenarios II and III. In scenario II, underestimation will be caused by intratumoral heterogeneity, and in scenario III, intertumoral heterogeneity caused by a dominant anterior Gleason score eight adenocarcinoma, wholly missed in the biopsy.

First, the material used in the puncture does not reflect a dominating tumour. The biopsy material in the second version does not contain a tissue piece of the dominant tumour, which may not reflect the complete volume of the pattern of 4 points on the Gleason scale. The material in the third variation has two fragments of patterns that do not entirely reflect the risk group of this malignancy. Both patterns are present in the fourth variety, fully reflecting the likelihood of illness progression. The patient is under active surveillance in the first choice (adenocarcinoma 6 (3+3) on the Gleason score) because most organ-limited malignancies on the Gleason score six are currently regarded clinically inconsequential [8].

When the valid Gleason score is known, radical treatment can be considered in the last three scenarios. Increased usage of high-resolution imaging during diagnostic biopsies. The ability to see prostate cancer's primary focus may help prevent biopsy errors. Prostate biopsy with tissue biomarker analysis may have the same sampling bias as histopathological analysis. Molecular heterogeneity in some but not all biomarkers may represent morphological intratumoral heterogeneity. Overexpression of the ETS-related gene (ERG) as a symptom of TMPRSS2-ERG fusions can occur in the early stages of prostate carcinogenesis and high-grade prostatic intraepithelial neoplasia. However, it is less common in metastatic prostate cancer than primary prostate cancer [9]. It could imply that TMPRSS2-ERG fusion occurs exceptionally early in prostate cancer, explaining its homogenous expression in most tumour foci, including those with a Gleason score of 7 points.

Sowalsky A.G. et al. study [10] directly confirmed the monoclonal character of such anatomically diverse tumour foci. A recent publication, in particular, showed that Gleason grade 4 cancer regions with cribriform development patterns contain the same TMPRSS2-ERG breakpoints as comparable Gleason grade 3 areas. Given the ad hoc nature of these breakpoints, this demonstrates the clonal similarity of grade 3 and 4 regions within the same tumour lesion.

The PTEN deletion had a more diversified pattern of genetic heterogeneity than TMPRSS2-ERG fusions in multifocal illness. The substantial interfocal mismatch for both TMPRSS2-ERG fusions and PTEN deletions, on the other hand, is consistent with the idea that several prostate cancer foci can originate independently in the same prostate gland and that individual tumour foci may have different genomic rearrangement patterns [11].

As a result, PTEN deletion or loss is frequently heterogeneous within a single tumour lesion (molecular intratumoral heterogeneity), with positive and negative tumour areas directly nearby. The PTEN deletion found in the grade 3 component was also present in the respective grade 4 adjacent component in two of four well-studied prostate cancers with a Gleason score of 7 (3+4) that were found to be monoclonal based on TMPRSS2-ERG breakpoint analysis as mentioned above [10]. In contrast, in the other two cases, only the grade 4 component showed a loss of PTEN. PTEN is more likely to be lost in prostate tumours with a Gleason score of 7 or higher than in pure tumours with a Gleason score 6 (3+3). The clinical significance of this finding may be that the presence of a PTEN deletion or loss in a biopsy with a Gleason score of 6 (3+3) may indicate the presence of a Gleason grade 4 that was not present in the biopsy due to sampling bias, or an increased likelihood of prostate cancer progression [10].

1.2. Analytical Capabilities of Tissue Biomarkers

Because of the small size of the sample and the usually partial involvement of the core of the biopsy by cancer, the use of prostate biopsy for the diagnosis of tissue biomarkers presents its technical hurdles. Modern techniques, such as the Nanostring technology [12], enable the precise measurement of individual messenger RNA (mRNA) molecules using only a tiny amount of RNA taken from formalin-fixed and paraffin-embedded biopsy tissue. When extracting DNA or RNA from prostate cancer, it is required to obtain optimal purity by labelling the carcinoma on traditional HE-stained slides, which can then be utilized as a template for dissecting the equivalent area on unstained paraffin sections. Using a set length of prostate core tissue to be extracted can help standardize the amount of dissected prostate cancer tissue. For example, mRNA isolation may necessitate at least 2 cm of prostate cancer tissue. When a defined cancer focus in a thick biopsy is a continuous track 5 mm long, four sections of 10 m are required, but two sections of 10 m are sufficient for a prostate cancer of 10 mm [13].

Most people with low-risk prostate cancer are now thought to be able to forego urgent treatment because their disease is generally indolent and not considered life-threatening [14]. Unfortunately, prostate biopsy sampling bias, combined with the heterogeneity of prostate cancer in an individual patient, might result in an underestimation of prostate cancer aggressiveness, which happens in approximately 20% of low-risk patients. Patients with intermediate-risk prostate cancer have cancer that, if left untreated, can progress to metastatic cancer but still have a window of opportunity for radical therapy. However, approximately 20-40% of individuals at intermediate risk do not respond to medication, and another 10-20% may not require therapy since their condition is inactive. Predictive biomarkers are thought to improve substratification in individuals, particularly in low and intermediate-risk categories.

There are several types of prostate cancer biomarkers (reviews are available in [15], including (1) susceptibility biomarkers that indicate an individual's risk of developing (potentially aggressive) prostate cancer, (2) diagnostic biomarkers that detect (potentially aggressive) prostate cancer glands, (3) predictive biomarkers that improve risk stratification, and (4) predictive biomarkers that identify patients who will benefit the most from specific treatments.

Most biomarkers are DNA polymorphisms discovered in germline DNA, frequently evaluated on peripheral blood leukocytes. However, diagnostic biomarkers can be proteins (e.g., PSA), (methylated) DNA (e.g., GSTP1 or TMPRSS2-ERG fusion gene), or RNA (e.g., PCA3) markers. In males with suspected prostate cancer, it is most commonly identified in blood or urine taken following prostate massage). Protein, RNA, or DNA alterations discovered in various sources of prostate tissue can be prognostic tissue biomarkers, but they can also be detected in the patient's blood or urine. They are most commonly found in specimens from prostatectomy or transurethral resection, but their most important application is in prostate needle biopsy material obtained prior to a specific treatment. This final tissue source will reduce the amount of cancer tissue accessible for biomarker testing.

In recent years, a slew of novel tissue biomarkers has emerged, intending to diagnose, stratify, and forecast disease risk at various stages of medical care. On the other hand, new, more accurate PCa biomarkers have enormous promise to enhance diagnosis, risk assessment, and prognosis. This knowledge reduces the number of needless surgical operations and more selective treatment of PCa patients (Table 1).

Table 1. Tissue markers for risk stratification in localized prostate cancer

Test Name	Manufacturer	Genetic material tested	Endpoint	Test Report	Target Population	Reference
Repeat Biopsy						
ConfirmMDx	MDxHealth	Methylation status of 3 genes (GSTP1, RASSF1, APC)	Risk of PCa on repeat biopsy	Likelihood of PCa in %	Men with negative biopsy and considering the second one	
After Biopsy: Active Surveillance vs. Intervention						
Prolaris Biopsy	Myriad Genetics	Expression levels (RNA) of 31 cell-cycle progression genes	The 10-year risk of PCa-specific mortality	CCP Score: 0-6	Men with PCa on biopsy	
Decipher Biopsy	GenomeDx Biosciences	Expression levels (RNA) of 22 genes (LASP1, IQGAP3, NFIB, S1PR4, THBS2, ANO7, PCDH7, MYBPC1, EPPK1, TS3P, PBX1, NUSAP1, ZWILCH, UBE2C, CAMK2N1, RABGAP1, PCAT-32, GLYATL1P4, PCAT-80, TNFRSF19)	5-year risk metastasis Likelihood of high-grade PCa on RP The 10-year risk of PCa-specific mortality	GC Score: 0-1.0	Men with localized PCa	
Oncotype DX	Genomic Health	Expression levels (RNA) of 12 genes (AZGP1, KLK2, SRD5A2, FAM13C, FLNC, GSN, TPM2, GSTM2, TPX2, BGN, COL1A1, SFRP4)	Likelihood of GGG 1 or GGG2 on RP Likelihood of organ confined PCa on RP	GPS Score: 0-100	Men with shallow- and low-risk PCa*	

Table 1. (Continued)

Test Name	Manufacturer	Genetic material tested	Endpoint	Test Report	Target Population	Reference
ProMark	Metamark	Quantitative levels of 8 proteins (DERL1, CUL2, SMAD4, PDSS2, HSPA9, FUS, pS6, YBOX1)	Risk of GGG ≥ 3 or non-organ confined PCa on RP	ProMark Score: 0-100	Men with GGG 1 or 2 on biopsy	
PTEN / TMPRSS2:ERG	Metamark	PTEN deletion and TMPRSS2:ERG fusion	-	Risk groups	Men with GGG 1 or 2 on biopsy	
Management after RP: Further Treatment vs. Observation						
Polaris	Myriad Genetics	Expression levels (RNA) of 31 cell-cycle progression genes	The 10-year risk of BCR	CCP Score: 0-6	Men after RP	
Decipher	GenomeDx Biosciences	Expression levels (RNA) of 22 genes 5-year risk of metastasis	The 10-year risk of PCa-specific mortality	GC Score: 0-1.0	Men with high-risk pathology or high-risk clinical features after RP	

* - PCa, prostate cancer; BCR, biochemical recurrence; CCP, cell cycle progression; GC, genomic classifier; GGG, Gleason grade group; GPS, genomic prostate score; RP, radical prostatectomy.

** - based on NCCN risk group.

Table 1 also elcited bias of sampling in case of puncture biopsy of the prostate (with patterns of presence of adenocarcinoma of the prostate 3 points on the Gleason scale and 4 points on the Gleason scale).

An ideal diagnostic biomarker has high specificity (the capacity of the test to identify persons without disease accurately; actual negative percentage), high sensitivity (the ability of the test to identify people with disease correctly; actual positive percentage), and simplified detection ease. This method's advantages are use, reproducibility, unambiguous recommendations for clinicians, cost-effectiveness, and quantitative results based on readily available body fluids or samples.

The genetic profile of solid tumours is currently retrieved through surgical or biopsy specimens; however, the latter treatment may only sometimes be performed frequently due to its intrusive nature. A single biopsy provides a geographically and temporally constrained view of the tumour that may not reflect its heterogeneity.

This study examines the present level of knowledge regarding available diagnostic and prognostic molecular markers for prostate cancer, as well as those in development, and assesses their clinical utility.

2.0. Tissue Biomarkers

2.1. PTEN/TMPRSS2:ERG

The traditional carcinogenesis model implies tumour formation during the clinical and pathological phases of the disease [16]. There is compelling evidence that genomic rearrangements are the initial event in oncogenesis.

The most prevalent genetic alteration in prostate cancer is the fusion of the ERG and TMPRSS2 genes. ERG is an oncogene that encodes a transcription factor from the ETS family. Other members of this gene family are rearranged and overexpressed in prostate cancer at a lower frequency. ERG overexpression in tissue, urine, and blood samples can be utilized to diagnose prostate cancer [17].

ERG was often overexpressed in prostate cancer in 2005 [18]. Tomlins S.A. et al. described the TMPRSS2-ERG chimeric gene, which results from the fusion of TMPRSS2 and ERG, in 2005. The mechanism behind this overexpression was discovered to be a recurrent genomic rearrangement between the initial exon(s) of the TMPRSS2 and ERG oncogenes (Figure 2) [19].

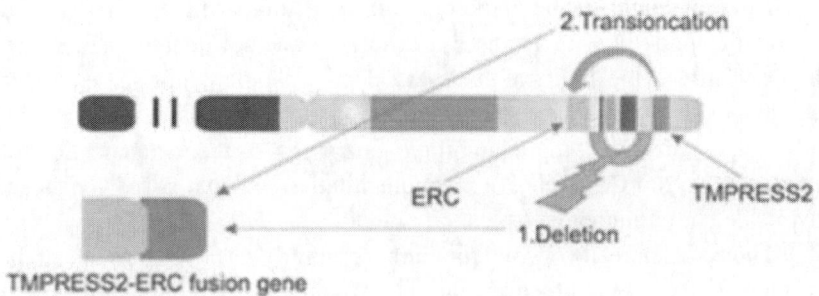

Figure 2. Schematic representation of the TMPRSS2-ERG fusion at chromosome region 21q22 [20].

TMPRSS2 at 21q22.3 and ERG at 21q22.2 are two fusion genes that map to chromosome 21. The loss of 2.8 Mb of genomic DNA between TMPRSS2 and ERG is the most common route of gene fusion [20]. A frequent chromosomal rearrangement in prostate cancer is the chemical gene TMPRSS2:ERG. Although the TMPRSS2:ERG fusion gene was not a valid predictor of biochemical recurrence or PCa-specific mortality, its presence was linked to a higher T-stage and a higher probability of metastasis [21]. According to particular research, prostate cancer fused to TMPRSS2:ERG contributes to a more aggressive cancer phenotype linked to a higher tumour stage and prostate cancer-specific mortality. Demichelis F. et al. discovered that the fusion transcript was related to metastasis and deadly prostate cancer in 252 patients under active surveillance for T1a-bNxM0 tumours with a mean follow-up of 9.1 years [22].

Without ERG fusion, homozygous or PTEN loss has been linked to PCa-specific mortality. This connection, however, was not observed in patients with PTEN loss due to ERG fusion. As a result, a TMPRSS2:ERG fusion may regulate the consequences of PTEN deficiency on disease biology [23].

PTEN is a tumour suppressor gene that regulates cell division by altering other proteins and lipids via phosphatase action. PTEN deficiency inhibits the PI3K signalling pathway, which regulates cell growth and proliferation. PTEN deficiency has been linked to high-grade malignancy, tumour growth, and poor prognosis in PCa [24]. TU. Ahearn et al. discovered that PTEN loss in the presence of TMPRSS2:ERG fusion is independently linked with PCa development [25].

PTEN/TMPRSS2:ERG study looks for both PTEN and TMPRSS2:ERG fusion genes in biopsy samples. PTEN deletion or TMPRSS2:ERG implies more aggressive PCa [26]. The effect of the PTEN/TMPRSS2:ERG tissue assay on therapeutic decision-making has yet to be investigated. The MyProstateScore test (LynxDx et al., MI, USA) is a new advancement that uses urine TMPRSS2:ERG, urinary PCa 3 antigen, and blood PSA to exclude grade 2 tumours in men who have not had biopsy [27].

PTEN/TMPRSS2:ERG is currently available as a stand-alone test for risk stratification for males with atypical illness, high-grade prostate neoplasia in situ, and individuals with grade 1 or 2 PCa. On the other hand, PTEN mutations and TMPRSS2:ERG fusions are frequently examined as part of commercially accessible Next Generation Sequencing (NGS) panels like FoundationOne CDx. The latter is the first FDA-approved tissue diagnostic complex (CDx) for all solid tumours that have been clinically and analytically verified. The PTEN/TMPRSS2:ERG assay is no longer recommended as a stand-alone test by the NCCN. However, NCCN recommendations currently recommend germline genetic testing for all men with high, very high-risk, regional, or metastatic PCa, as well as men with PCa who have Ashkenazi Jewish ancestry or a family history of high-risk germline mutations (e.g., BRCA1/2, Lynch syndrome). Furthermore, men with PCa with a positive family history of cancer (a brother or father or numerous family members with PCa under 60 or more than three tumours on one side of the family) should have germline genetic testing [28].

2.2. Decipher

The DecipherTM Comprehensive genetic Test (GenomeDx, San Diego, CA, USA) is a genetic test created in collaboration between GenomeDx Biosciences (Vancouver, British Columbia, Canada) and the Mayo Clinic (Rochester, Minnesota, USA) to predict the course of disease following major surgery. In men with high-risk or disease progression following radical prostatectomy, the Decipher test predicts the risk of metastasis up to 5 years after RP and prostate cancer death up to 10 years. 22 RNAs are analyzed on microarrays to analyze the expression of 22 genes ((LASP1, IQGAP3, NFIB, S1PR4, THBS2, ANO7, PCDH7, MYBPC1, EPPK1, TSBP, PBX1, NUSAP1). ZWILCH, UBE2C, CAMK2N1, RABGAP1, PCAT-32, GLYATL1P4, PCAT-80, TNFRSF19) [29].

These genes involve various biological activities, including cell proliferation, differentiation, adhesion, cell cycle development, and androgen receptor signalling [30]. To conduct the investigation, RNA can be extracted from formalin-fixed paraffin-embedded tissue and a tumour sample no smaller than 0.5 mm in size [31]. In comparison tests, the test performed exceptionally well in predicting metastases (AUC, 0.75-0.83) and cancer mortality (AUC 0.78) and outperformed the physical characteristics of the prostate tumour (AUC 0.69) [32].

For the next five years, the Decipher test is approved for predicting the development of metastases [33]. Furthermore, based on the results of this test, it was possible to estimate when postoperative radiation (adjuvant) should be performed. DecipherTM is also the sole independent predictor of metastasis development in patients with biochemical recurrence following surgery.

Alshalalfa M. et al. [34] investigated differences between patients who acquired BCR, clinical metastases, or did not have any poor outcomes throughout follow-up and discovered that DecipherTM could be a beneficial tool for better patient prognosis. This study discovered that disease-free and BCR-only patients had identical transcription patterns, unlike individuals who acquired metastases and displayed a distinct transcription profile that may be detected in a primary tumour/PCa sample. These findings were verified in 219 patients with high-risk PCa treated with RP at the Mayo Clinic. Higher GS scores were the most predictive of metastasis development in multivariate analysis [35].

Klein et al., for example, discovered that the Decipher score from prostate biopsy specimens strongly predicted metastasis up to 10 years after RP, with an AUC of 0.8 [36].

We used validated clinical and genetic risk stratification to predict survival after RP. Klein [37] and Cooperberg M.R. [38] described an improvement in the prediction of clinical outcomes following RP by incorporating verified clinical parameters and DecipherTM scores in the same data. Model.

The AUC in predicting metastases for DecipherTM, the generally used Stevenson model clinical scores, and the Prostate Cancer Risk Rating Scale (CAPRA-S) were 77%, 75%, and 72%, respectively. When DecipherTM was added to the Stevenson nomogram, the AUC increased to 79%. Similar findings were provided for cancer mortality (CSM) following RP; the AUCs for CAPRA-S and DecipherTM were 75% and 78%, respectively. Patients with high GC and CAPRA-S risk scores were at the most significant risk of acquiring CSM. Furthermore, DecipherTM was reclassified, allowing patients to be less concerned.

Furthermore, Lobo et al. [39] found that using the DecipherTM test in the postoperative phase increased quality-adjusted life expectancy (QALY). In several investigations, the authors concluded that Decipher was an independent predictor of unfavourable pathology, biochemical failure, metastasis, malignancy, and overall survival. Decipher is more beneficial for intermediate-risk PCa as well as decision-making after prostatectomy.

The National Comprehensive Cancer Network (NCCN) recommends that men with a very low, low, or intermediate biopsy risk of PCa and a life expectancy of at least ten years be offered the Decipher test. In this context, the goal of the test is to assist in selecting individuals for active surveillance. Following prostatectomy, men with pT2 disease with a positive surgical margin or any pT3 disease may be administered the Decipher test to help decide whether to undergo adjuvant radiotherapy [28].

2.3. Prolaris Molecular Score (Myriad Genetics) v3.0

The Prolaris Molecular Score test (Myriad Genetics, Salt Lake City, Utah, USA) assesses the expression of 31 genes (FOXM1, ASPM, TK1, PRC1, CDC20, BUB1B, PBK, DTL, CDKN3, RRM2, ASF1B, CEP55, CDC2, DLGAP5, C18orf24, RAD51, KIF11, BIRC5, RAD54L, CENPM, KIAA0101, KIF20A, PTTG1, CDCA8, NUSAP1, PLK1, CDCA3, ORC6L, CENPF, TOP2A, MCM10) cell cycle progression score (CCP) associated with cancer proliferation and can be performed either on a biopsy or a RP specimen [40].

The CCP score is between 0 and 10, with a higher score indicating more aggressive cancer and a higher probability of disease progression [41]. Each unit increase represents a doubling of gene expression, indicating a more aggressive tumour. Men with freshly diagnosed PCa (Prolaris biopsy test) and men who had already undergone a prostatectomy (Prolaris post-prostatectomy test) were given the CCP score. The Prolaris biopsy test indicates a 10-year risk of PCa mortality and metastasis with radical treatment, whereas the Prolaris test following prostatectomy indicates a 10-year chance of biochemical recurrence.

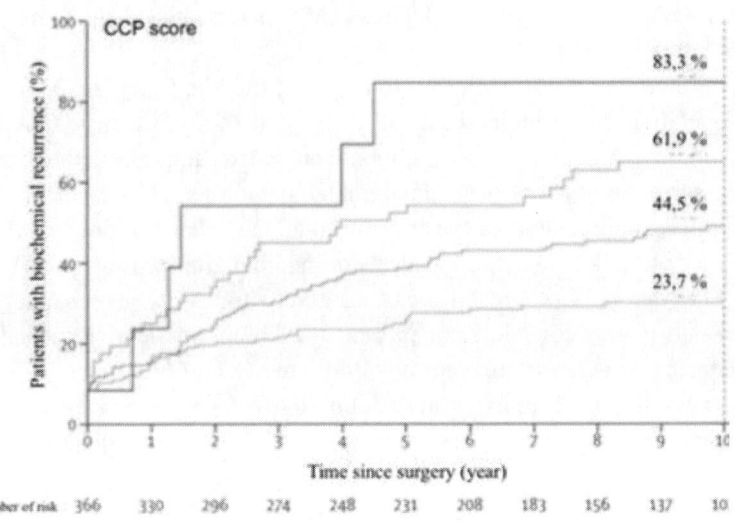

Figure 3. Analytical capabilities of the Prolaris test in the radical prostatectomy cohort.

The Prolaris study comprises a 31-gene index representing the whole collection of CCP genes best reliably uncovered. The predictive value of this gene signature was first described in a retrospective study that found a significant correlation between CCP score and clinical outcomes in two separate cohorts: 366 patients undergoing surgery and 337 men with localized PCa diagnosed by transurethral resection and treated conservatively. The CCP score was linked with the likelihood of biochemical recurrence (RR 1.77, 95% CI 1.40-2.22, P 0.001) in the prostatectomy cohort and specific mortality from PCa (RR 2.57, 95% CI 1.93- 3.43, P 0.001) in the PCa group. The CCP scale's predictive usefulness was initially revealed in a 2011 article in which the authors employed two separate patient groups for a valid assessment [42].

The first group included 366 patients who underwent RP, while the second group included 337 men who had conservative treatment after being identified with clinically localized prostate cancer via transurethral resection (TURP). CCP was linked with the probability of biochemical recurrence (HR 1.77, 95% CI 1.40-2.22, P 0.001) in the prostatectomy cohort and specific mortality from PCa (HR 2.57, 95% CI 1.93-3.43, P 0.001) in the conservatively treated cohort in this analysis [42].

The Prolaris biopsy test may help men decide between active surveillance and localized treatment (surgery or radiation therapy). Bischoff et al.

examined CCP in 582 men undergoing radical prostatectomy. They found that an increase in biopsy CCP was associated with biochemical recurrence (RR per unit estimate 1.47, 95% CI 1.23-1, 76, P 0.001) and metastasis progression (HR per assessment unit 4.19, 95% CI 2.08-8.45, P 0.001) [43].

Kuzik et al. found that biopsy CCP was an independent predictor of prostate cancer-specific death (RR per unit 1.76, 95% CI 1.44- 2.14, P0.001) after controlling for Gleason score, PSA, disease grade, and clinical stage in a sample of 585 regularly monitored men in 2015 [44]. By integrating the patient's PSA, clinical stage, % positive, biopsy grade group, and AUA risk group, the Prolaris biopsy test also delivers a 10-year specific mortality risk from PCa [45].

CCP examination resulted in a change in treatment for 47.8% of patients, according to PROCEDE-1000, an extensive prospective registry with approximately 1600 participants [46]. In particular, 75% of cases had their treatment de-escalated, while 25% had their treatment intensified. Despite its usage as a tool to assist doctors and patients in making tailored treatment decisions, no prospective data have demonstrated the therapeutic superiority of the decisions on which the test is based.

De Pouvourville (no full text) presented the cost-effectiveness of MMR in low-risk localized prostate cancer as a conference abstract and discovered that including MMR in the initial risk stratification would save €1,709 over the patient's lifetime and improve quality of life by avoiding complications associated with radical treatment [47]. The present test assigns a risk score from 0 to 10, with higher scores indicating more aggressive malignancies. When paired with clinical features, the test indicates the chance of metastases and mortality ten years after final therapy.

The present test assigns a risk score from 0 to 10, with higher scores corresponding to more aggressive malignancies. When paired with clinical features, the test reports the risk of metastasis ten years after final therapy and the probability of death mouth ten years after final treatment. A Prolaris biopsy may be suggested by the NCCN recommendations [28] for men with extremely low, low, or favourable intermediate biopsy-risk PCa and a life expectancy of at least ten years.

2.4. Oncotype DX

Oncotype DX (Genomic Health, Redwood City, CA, USA) is a prostate biopsies-based RNA expression assay. We wanted to see if using GPS was connected with an increased incidence of unfavourable outcomes in men who were on active monitoring and later had radical prostatectomy. The polymerase chain reaction reverse transcription operations were used to analyze the mRNA expression of 17 genes (AZGP1, KLK2, SRD5A2, RAM13C, FLNC, GSN, TPM2, GSTM2, TPX2, BGN, BGN, COL1A1, SFRP4, ARF1, ATP5E, CLTC, GPS1, PGK1) in prostate samples (Figure 4).

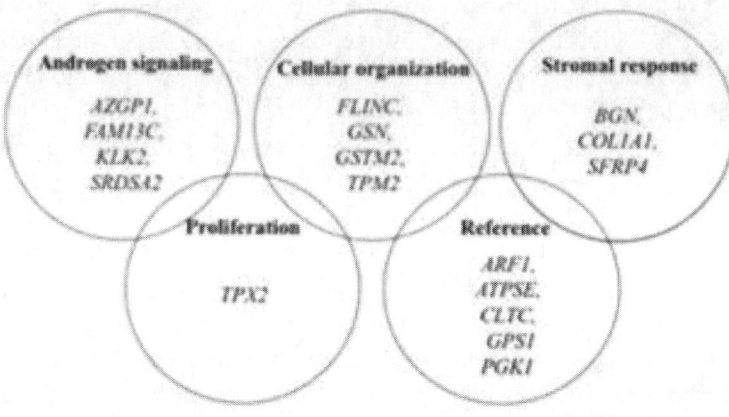

Figure 4. Genes included in the Oncotype DX® Prostate Genomic Assay.

These genes are combined to compute the prostate genome scale (GPS), which ranges from 0 to 100. GPS predicts the chance of an unfavourable form of the illness in patients who have had radical prostatectomy, active surveillance, or rapid prostatectomy. A high GPS score is linked to an increased risk of illness progression [48].

The analysis can be interpreted in four ways: (1) predicting aggressive prostate cancer clinical recurrence (local recurrence and metastatic disease) and other endpoints, (2) predicting aggressive prostate cancer based on tumour heterogeneity and multifocality (3) higher expression of stromal genes responsiveness and proliferation was linked to more aggressive prostate cancer, (4) higher expression of cell organization genes and androgens was linked to less aggressive prostate cancer.

2.5. Application Indications

The Oncotype DX prostate cancer test is recommended for men diagnosed with very low, low, or intermediate risk NCCN prostate cancer and is a candidate for active surveillance. Only individuals at intermediate risk regarded as potential candidates for active surveillance (see features below) are considered suitable for examination. Several primary treatment options are described in the NCCN guidelines for people with clinically low-risk prostate cancer. The primary treatment option chosen for each patient should be based on the patient's life expectancy and the risk of recurrence evaluation. The NCCN recommendations (Table 2) specify relapse risk staging systems.

Table 2. Risk categories based on NCCN® (2023)

Very Low	Low	Intermediate
T1c	T1 – T2a	T2b – T2c or
Gleason score ≤ 6	Gleason score ≤ 6	Gleason score 7
PSA < 10 ng/ml	PSA < 10 ng/ml	PSA < 10-20 ng/ml
Fewer than three prostate biopsy cores positive, ≤ 50% cancer in each core		
PSA density < 0,15 ng/mL/g		

Clinicopathological parameters of patients, such as tumour size, Gleason score 3, PSA levels, number of positive biopsies, fraction of malignant tissue in biopsies, and PSA density, are used to stage risk.

The most recent NCCN guidelines accept tissue-based molecular genetic testing as a risk stratification option for men with localized prostate cancer with a life expectancy of more than five years.

Clinical validation From 1997 to 2011, 395 individuals with early-stage prostate cancer underwent radical prostatectomy at the University of California, San Francisco [49] (low/low average risk).

Patients were ruled out of the trial if they had any of the following conditions: (1) biopsy Gleason score > 3+4, (2) biopsy Gleason score 3+4 with substantial disease volume, (3) clinically advanced disease or lesion lymph nodes, (4) PSA >20, (5) tissue absence or insufficiency (tumour length at biopsy 1 mm), or 6) absence of RP or biopsy for central analysis. Within six months after the initial biopsy, all patients underwent radical prostatectomy.

GPS was a statistically significant predictor of Gleason 4+3 or higher pathology or non-organ disease (p=0.002). The analysis predicted high-grade illness (primary Gleason 4/5) and pT3 disease with ORs of 2.5 (1.6-3.9) and

2.2 (1.5-2.3), respectively, for every 20 units of analysis score rise in a pre-specified binary logistic regression analysis with Gleason score control. The researchers concluded that Oncotype DX GPS provides independent predictive information in addition to all usual clinical and pathological data [49].

According to Klein et al. and colleagues' research, the prostate genome score (GPS) is a statistically significant predictor of unfavourable pathology, defined as a Gleason score of 4+3 or above, and non-organ disease (p=0.002). The study predicted high-grade illness (primary Gleason 4/5) or pT3 disease with ORs of 2.5 (1.6-3.9) and 2.2 (1.5-2.3), respectively, with an increase for every 20 units of the analytical scale in a pre-specified binary logistic regression analysis with Gleason score control. The researchers found that the Oncotype DX GPS test and other traditional clinical and morphological characteristics provide independent predictive information [49].

Cullen J. and colleagues investigated the predictive capability of biochemical relapse (BCR) and Oncotype DX (HR/20 GPS units = 2.9; 95% CI: 2.0, 4.2; p0.001), (2) re-validated as a strong and independent predictor of unfavourable pathology (AP) during surgery. (3) substantially related to metastasis (HR/20 GPS units = 3.8; 95% CI: 1.1, 12.6; p 0.001). The researchers found that because GPS is associated with immediate and long-term clinical outcomes, this analysis represents a credible independent predictor of PCa aggressiveness. In this equal access healthcare system, GPS-measured tumour aggressiveness and outcomes were comparable in African-American and Caucasian men [50].

According to NCCN+GPS, four out of five patients with very low-risk prostate cancer will have favourable pathology during prostatectomy. In comparison, no more than two out of three patients with intermediate-risk prostate cancer will have favourable pathology. The Oncotype DX test results for prostate cancer should be interpreted with NCCN guidelines and other laboratory and clinical data available to the clinician [28].

2.6. ConfirmMDx

ConfirmMDx (MDxHealth, Inc., Irvine, CA, USA) is a multiplex epigenetic tissue analysis intended to stratify individuals being considered for a repeat prostate biopsy. This test measures the methylation of the promoter regions of three tumour suppressor genes: Pi1 glutathione S-transferase domain family (GSTP1), adenomatous polyposis Coli (APC), and Ras association

(RalGDS/AF-6). 2 (RASSF2) gene in benign changes in prostate biopsy tissue samples [51]. These epigenetic alterations are frequently observed in PCa. This test aims to detect a "halo" effect, which is an area around a PC lesion that may appear normal morphologically but has epigenetic changes consistent with malignancy. There is an elevated risk of PCa when CpG islands proliferate in the promoter regions of these genes. According to the theory, the normal prostate tissue surrounding the cancer will undergo epigenetic alterations [52].

The novel ConfirmMDx test (1) detects men who are not at risk of developing prostate cancer and eliminates unnecessary biopsies. Determine which patients (2) require therapy. It also aids in the identification of high-risk patients for further examination or therapy [53]. Up to 30 months after the initial biopsy, the test has a 90% negative predictive value and is regarded as the most significant predictor of biopsy outcomes [54].

ConfirmMDx may be considered an option for people planning a repeat biopsy because this test may identify people at a higher risk of being diagnosed with prostate cancer on repeat biopsy. MolDX approves this assay for limited coverage to reduce unnecessary repeat prostate biopsies. Many men with an initial negative biopsy due to an elevated PSA will undergo additional biopsies. Based on the presence of genomic halo effects in histologically normal PCa adjacent to cancerous lesions, the ConfirmMDx assay (MDx Health, Irvine, CA) measures GSTP1, APC, RASSF1 methylation levels in pathologically benign biopsy specimens to determine the risk of subsequent PCa detection [55].

The MATLOC study demonstrated that ConfirmMDx has a sensitivity and specificity of 68% and 64%, respectively, for detecting occult PCa, defined as a negative biopsy followed by a positive biopsy within 30 months. In addition, ConfirmMDx has been shown to reduce unnecessary prostate biopsies by up to 64% [56]. The NPV was 90% (95% confidence interval, 87-93%). ConfirmMDx predicted patient outcome in multivariate analysis (OR 3.17; 95% CI 1.81-5.53). In the United States, a comparable validation study was conducted utilizing archival tissue from 350 biopsy-negative individuals who underwent repeat biopsies within 24 months [57]. The NPV was 88% (95% confidence interval, 85%-91%), and the test was repeated. In multivariate analysis, they appeared to predict outcomes (OR 2.69; 95% CI 1.60-4.51). The sensitivity and specificity of the assay for detecting subsequent PCa were 68% and 64%, with a negative predictive value (NPV) of 90% (95% CI 87–93%) [56].

In a 2018 review article by G. Gurioli et al., the sensitivity and specificity of the ConfirmMDx prostate biopsy test for the detection of prostate cancer were 81.7% and 95.8%, respectively [58]. According to the DOCUMENT study, ConfirmMDx is an independent predictor of PC compared to other clinicopathological characteristics, with a negative predictive value of about 90% [54]. Furthermore, Van Neste L. et al. discovered that men with low DNA methylation levels in benign biopsies have a 96% negative predictive value for high-grade cancer [57]. Regarding the role of ConfirmMDx in clinical decision-making, Wonju et al. discovered that only 4.4% of ConfirmMDx-negative males received repeat biopsies, compared to 43% in the PLCO research [59]. All repeat biopsies of patients who tested negative for ConfirmMDx were likewise negative in our research. Furthermore, Van Neste et al. demonstrated that by using a probability threshold of 15%, 30 needless repeat biopsies per 100 patients can be avoided [57].

The National Comprehensive Cancer Network (NCCN) recommends this test for males who have had at least one negative biopsy in the past [28].

2.7. ProMark

The ProMark test (Metamark, Cambridge, Massachusetts, USA) is a protein-based assay that quantifies the levels of eight proteins in a prostate biopsy material (DERL1, CUL2, SMAD4, PDSS2, HSPA9, FUS, pS6, and YBOX1). Immunofluorescence. These proteins are essential in cell signalling, stress response, and cell proliferation [60, 61]. Metamark Genetics' Promark score is the first reported protein biomarker to measure prostate cancer risk. It has been created explicitly for use in prostate biopsy specimens and to address issues related to sampling mistakes in prostate biopsy samples. It is built on the Quantitative Multiplex Immunofluorescence (QMPI) platform, which examines eight protein-based indicators [62].

Protein evaluation is predicated on the considerable intratumoral heterogeneity that characterizes PCa. As a result, the protein-based panel strives to give information collected from the most aggressive cells in a tumour. The benefit of using a protein marker over a genomic marker in prostate biopsy specimens is that genetic markers require an experienced pathologist to look for the highest-grade prostate cancer (subjective assessment). In contrast, proteomics can detect high-grade molecular features even in small tissue samples containing varying amounts of cancerous and non-cancerous tissues (objective assessment). The test differentiated between men with favourable (surgical GS 3 + 4 = 7 and organ-restricted disease) and unfavourable (surgical GS 7, non-organ disease) pathology in a validation trial of 276 men with matching biopsies and RP. At the same time, the autonomous test's AUC was 0.68 [63].

ProMark assigns a score from 0 to 1, indicating the risk of Gleason disease 4 + 3 or non-organ disease in RP. The test is indicated for males at very low or low risk of NCCN and considering starting active monitoring. A good biomarker risk score is defined as 0.33 on a scale of 0 to 1, and an unfavourable biomarker as >0.80. The predictive values for favourable pathology in the shallow and low-risk NCCN groups and the low-risk D'Amico groups were 95%, 81.5%, and 87.2%, respectively, with a risk score of 0.33, more significant than the present risk. The classification categories themselves (80.3%, 63.8%, and 70.6%). However, the predictive value of unfavourable pathology was 76.9% in all risk groups when the risk index was more significant than 0.80. The validation research achieved two primary endpoints: benign pathology vs unfavourable pathology (AUC, 0.68; P0.0001; OR 20.9) and GS 6 pathology versus GS 6 pathology (AUC, 0.65; P0.0001; OR 12.95) [63].

This marker is still in the process of being validated. It was discovered that a "favourable" score of 0.33 predicted favourable pathology in 95% of deficient-risk patients and 81.5% of low-risk NCCN patients. The predictive value of unfavourable pathology was 76.9% in all risk categories, with biomarker risk scores greater than 0.8. In addition, the scientists conducted a validation analysis on 276 patients. They discovered that an eight-protein biomarker distinguishes benign from unfavourable illness and disease with a Gleason score of 6 and disease not associated with a Gleason score of 6 (AUC 0.68 and 0.65, respectively). The signature was then refined to include eight protein markers [63] with a score (0-1) that reflects the risk of unfavourable pathology in RP.

A score of less than 33 suggested a benign disease (90% sensitivity), whereas a score of more than 80 indicated an unpleasant pathology (95% specificity). It was discovered that increasing the Promark score by 25 points increases the chance of unfavourable pathology by 3.1-fold. When the NCCN risk criteria were included with the score, the AUC increased from 0.68 to 0.75. Saad et al. studied the relationship of Promark score in prostate biopsy with BCR and time to metastasis after RP in participants from a previously validated study. A score of more than 66 was highly related to BCR (HR 4.7) [64].

A randomized clinical trial assessing utility among 129 urologists using simulated cases of GG1 and GG2 in a before and after model discovered that a urologist told about the Promark test made 28.9% fewer active treatment recommendations based on results. Low and F-IR prostate cancer tests [65]. The Promark® score is between 0 and 100, with a higher score indicating more aggressive and fatal prostate cancer. It also forecasts BCR and metastases following RP.

ProMark is suggested by NCCN guidelines for men with extremely low or low biopsy-risk PCa and a life expectancy of at least ten years [28].

Conclusion

Prostate cancer is a hormone-dependent tumour with multifocal proliferation and intratumoral heterogeneity. The course of the disease and prognostic variations are determined by substantial genomic, epigenetic, and proteomic heterogeneity. Patients at risk with the same morphological pattern (Gleason score) may have significantly varied prognoses due to distinct genetic profiles [66].

In recent years, a slew of novel tissue biomarkers has emerged, intending to diagnose, stratify, and forecast disease risk at various stages of medical care. Tissue markers are used in everyday practice and have a place in prostate cancer therapy and diagnostic algorithms, as evidenced by publications and presentations in clinical recommendations. Tissue markers are an appropriate tool for risk assessment, prediction, and treatment with the goal of precision medicine, driven by increased knowledge of genomes and proteomics.

References

[1] Hyuna S., Jacques F., Rebecca L., Siegel, M. L., Isabelle S., Ahmedin J., Freddie B. (2021) Global Cancer Statistics 2020: GLOBOCAN Estimates of Incidence and Mortality Worldwide for 36 Cancers in 185 Countries. *CA Cancer J Clin.* 71(3):209-249. doi: 10.3322/caac.21660.

[2] Diamantis A., Magiorkinis E., Koutselini H. Fine-needle aspiration (FNA) biopsy: historical aspects. (2009) Folia Histochem. *Cytobiol.* 47,191–197.

[3] Alessandro C., Matteo S., Luciano B., Scarpelli M., Mazzucchelli R., Galosi A. B., Cheng L., Lopez-Beltran A., Briganti A., Montorsi F., Montironi R. (2017) Update on histopathological evaluation of lymphadenectomy specimens from prostate cancer patients. *World J Urol.* 35(4):517-526. doi: 10.1007/s00345-015-1752-8.

[4] Gerlinger M., Rowan A. J., Horswell S., Math M., Larkin J., Endesfelder D., Gronroos E., Martinez P., Matthews N., Stewart A., Tarpey P., Varela I., Phillimore B., Begum S., McDonald N. Q., Butler A., Jones D., Raine K., Latimer C., Santos C. R., Nohadani M., Eklund A. C., Spencer-Dene B., Clark G., Pickering L., Stamp G., Gore M., Szallasi Z., Downward J., Futreal P. A., Swanton C. Intratumor heterogeneity and branched evolution revealed by multi-region sequencing. (2012) *N. Engl. J. Med.* 366, 883–892.

[5] D'Amico A. V., Moul J., Carroll P. R., Sun L., Lubeck D., Chen M. H. (2003) Cancer-specific mortality after surgery or radiation for patients with clinically localized prostate cancer managed during the prostate-specific antigen era. *J Clin Oncol.* 21(11):2163–2172.

[6] Wolters T., Montironi R., Mazzucchelli R., Scarpelli M., Roobol M. J., van den Bergh R. C., van Leeuwen P. J., Hoedemaeker R. F., van Leenders G. J., Schröder F. H., van der Kwast T. H. (2012) Comparison of incidentally detected prostate cancer with screen-detected prostate cancer treated by prostatectomy. *Prostate.* 72(1):108–115.

[7] Guo C. C., Wang Y., Xiao L., Troncoso P., Czerniak B. A. (2012) The relationship of TMPRSS2-ERG gene fusion between primary and metastatic prostate cancers. *Hum Pathol.* 43(5):644–649.

[8] Van der Kwast T. H., Roobol M. J. (2013) Defining the threshold for significant versus insignificant prostate cancer. *Nat Rev Urol.* 10(8):473–482.

[9] Scheble V. J., Scharf G., Braun M., Ruiz C., Stürm S., Petersen K., Beschorner R., Bachmann A., Zellweger T., Fend F., Kristiansen G., Bubendorf L., Wernert N., Adler D., Perner S. (2012) ERG rearrangement in local recurrences compared to distant metastases of castration-resistant prostate cancer. *Virchows Arch.* 461(2):157–162.

[10] Sowalsky A. G., Ye H., Bubley G. J., Balk S. P. (2013) Clonal progression of prostate cancers from Gleason grade 3 to grade 4. *Cancer Res.* 73(3):1050–1055.

[11] Yoshimoto M., Ding K., Sweet J. M., Ludkovski O., Trottier G., Song K. S., Joshua A. M., Fleshner N. E., Squire J. A., Evans A. J., (2013) PTEN losses exhibit heterogeneity in multifocal prostatic adenocarcinoma and are associated with higher Gleason grade. *Mod Pathol.* 26(3): 435–447.

[12] Reis P. P., Waldron L., Goswami R. S., Xu W., Xuan Y., Perez-Ordonez B., Gullane P., Irish J., Jurisica I., Kamel-Reid S. (2011) mRNA transcript quantification in archival samples using multiplexed, colour-coded probes. *BMC Biotechnol.* 11:46.

[13] Freedland S. J., Gerber L., Reid J., Welbourn W., Tikishvili E., Park J., Younus A., Gutin A., Sangale Z., Lanchbury J. S., Salama J. K., Stone S. (2013) Prognostic utility of cell cycle progression score in men with prostate cancer after primary external beam radiation therapy. *Int J Radiat Oncol Biol Phys.* 86(5):848–853.

[14] Klotz L. (2013) Active surveillance: patient selection. *Curr Opin Urol.* 23(3):239–244.

[15] Choudhury A. D., Eeles R., Freedland S. J., Isaacs W. B., Pomerantz M. M., Schalken J. A., Tammela T. L., Visakorpi T. (2012) The role of genetic markers in the management of prostate cancer. *Eur Urol* 62(4):577–587.

[16] Stratton M. R., Campbell P. J., Futreal P. A. (2009) The cancer genome. *Nature.* 458:719–724.

[17] Qu X., Randhawa G., Friedman C., O'Hara-Larrivee S., Kroeger K., Dumpit R., True L., Vakar-Lopez F., Porter C., Vessella R., Nelson P., Fang M. (2013) A novel four-color fluorescence in situ hybridization assay for the detection of TMPRSS2 and ERG rearrangements in prostate cancer. *Cancer Genet.* 206: 1–11.

[18] Petrovics G., Liu A., Shaheduzzaman S., Furusato B., Sun C., Chen Y., Nau M., Ravindranath L., Chen Y., Dobi A., Srikantan V., Sesterhenn I. A., McLeod D. G., Vahey M., Moul J. W., Srivastava S. (2005) Frequent overexpression of ETS-related gene-1 (ERG1) in prostate cancer transcriptome. *Oncogene.* 24 3847–3852. doi:10.1038/sj.onc.1208518.

[19] Tomlins S. A., Rhodes D. R., Perner S., Dhanasekaran S. M., Mehra R., Sun X. W., Varambally S., Cao X., Tchinda J., Kuefer R., Lee C., Montie J. E., Shah R. B., Pienta K. J., Rubin M. A., Chinnaiyan A. M. (2005) Recurrent fusion of TMPRSS2 and ETS transcription factor genes in prostate cancer. *Science.* 310 644–648. doi:10.1126/science.1117679.

[20] Perner S., Demichelis F., Beroukhim R., Schmidt F. H., Mosquera J. M., Setlur S., Tchinda J., Tomlins S. A., Hofer M. D., Pienta K. G., Kuefer R., Vessella R., Sun X. W., Meyerson M., Lee C., Sellers W. R., Chinnaiyan A. M., Rubin M. A. (2006) TMPRSS2:ERG fusion-associated deletions provide insight into the heterogeneity of prostate cancer. *Cancer Res.* 66:8337.

[21] Song C, Chen H. (2018) Predictive Significance of TMRPSS2-ERG Fusion in Prostate Cancer: A Meta-Analysis. *Cancer Cell Int.* 18:177. doi: 10.1186/s12935-018-0672-2.

[22] Demichelis F., Fall K., Perner S., Andrén O., Schmidt F., Setlur S. R., Hoshida Y., Mosquera J. M., Pawitan Y., Lee C., Adami H. O., Mucci L. A., Kantoff P. W., Andersson S. O., Chinnaiyan A. M., Johansson J. E., Rubin M. A. (2007) TMPRSS2: ERG gene fusion associated with lethal prostate cancer in a watchful waiting cohort. *Oncogene.* 26:4596.

[23] Clinton T. N., Bagrodia A., Lotan Y., Margulis V., Raj G. V., Woldu S. L. (2017) Tissue-Based Biomarkers in Prostate Cancer. *Expert Rev Precis Med Drug Dev.* 2(5):249–60. doi: 10.1080/23808993.2017.1372687.

[24] Bertram J., Peacock J. W., Fazli L., Mui A. L., Chung S. W., Cox M. E., Monia B., Gleave M. E., Ong C. J. (2006) Loss of PTEN is Associated With Progression to Androgen Independence. *Prostate.* 66(9):895–902. doi:10.1002/pros.20411.

[25] Ahearn T. U., Pettersson A., Ebot E. M., Gerke T., Graff R. E., Morais C. L., Hicks J. L., Wilson K. M., Rider J. R., Sesso H. D., Fiorentino M., Flavin R., Finn S., Giovannucci E. L., Loda M., Stampfer M. J., De Marzo A. M., Mucci L. A., Lotan T. L. (2016) A Prospective Investigation of PTEN Loss and ERG Expression in Lethal Prostate Cancer. *J Natl Cancer Inst.* 108(2):djv346. doi: 10.1093/jnci/djv346.

[26] Jamaspishvili T., Berman D. M., Ross A. E., Scher H. I., De Marzo A. M., Squire J. A., Lotan T. L. (2018) Clinical Implications of PTEN Loss in Prostate Cancer. *Nat Rev Urol.* 15(4):222–34. doi: 10.1038/nrurol.2018.9.

[27] Tosoian J. J., Trock B. J., Morgan T. M., Salami S. S., Tomlins S. A., Spratt D. E., Siddiqui J., Kunju L. P., Botbyl R., Chopra Z., Pandian B., Eyrich N. W., Longton

G., Zheng Y., Palapattu G. S., Wei J. T., Niknafs Y. S., Chinnaiyan A. M. (2021) Use of the MyProstateScore Test to Rule Out Clinically Significant Cancer: Validation of a Straightforward Clinical Testing Approach. *J Urol.* 205(3):732–9. doi: 10.1097/JU.0000000000001430.

[28] National Comprehensive Cancer Network. *Guidelines Prostate Cancer V. 2.2023* – WebEx on June 12, 2023. (2023).

[29] Sharma N., Baruah M. M. (2019) The microRNA signatures: aberrantly expressed miRNAs in prostate cancer. *Clin Transl Oncol.* 21(2):126–144. doi:10.1007/s12094-018-1910-8.

[30] Erho N., Crisan A., Vergara I. A., Mitra A. P., Ghadessi M., Buerki C., Bergstralh E. J., Kollmeyer T., Fink S., Haddad Z., Zimmermann B., Sierocinski T., Ballman K. V., Triche T. J., Black P. C., Karnes R. J., Klee G., Davicioni E., Jenkins R. B. (2013) Discovery and Validation of a Prostate Cancer Genomic Classifier That Predicts Early Metastasis Following Radical Prostatectomy. *PLoS One.* 8(6):e66855. doi:10.1371/journal.pone.0066855 .

[31] Decipher Biosciences. (2021). Available at: https://decipherbio.com/wp-content/themes/decipher/assets/pdf/decipher-prostate-specimen-preparation-shipping-Instructions.pdf .

[32] Klein E. A., Haddad Z., Yousefi K., Lam L. L. C., Wang Q., Choeurng V., Palmer-Aronsten B., Buerki C., Davicioni E., Li J., Kattan M. W., Stephenson A. J., Magi-Galluzzi C. (2016) Decipher Genomic Classifier Measured on Prostate Biopsy Predicts Metastasis Risk. *Urology.* Apr;90:148–152. doi: 10.1016/j.urology. 2016.01.012.

[33] Nguyen P. L., Haddad Z., Ross A. E., Martin N. E., Deheshi S., Lam L. L. C., Chelliserry J., Tosoian J. J., Lotan T. L., Spratt D. E., Stoyanova R. S., Punnen S., Ong K., Buerki C., Aranes M., Kolisnik T., Margrave J., Yousefi K., Choeurng V., Davicioni E., Trock B. J., Kane C. J., Pollack A., Davis J. W., Feng F. Y., Klein E. A. (2017) Ability of a Genomic Classifier to Predict Metastasis and Prostate Cancer-specific Mortality after Radiation or Surgery based on Needle Biopsy Specimens. *Eur Urol.* Nov;72(5):845–852. doi: 10.1016/j.eururo.2017.05.009.

[34] Alshalalfa M., Crisan A., Vergara I. A., Ghadessi M., Buerki C., Erho N., Yousefi K., Sierocinski T., Haddad Z., Black P. C., Karnes R. J., Jenkins R. B., Davicioni E. (2015) Clinical and genomic analysis of metastatic prostate cancer progression with a background of postoperative biochemical recurrence. *BJU Int.* 116:556–67. doi:10.1111/bju.13013.

[35] Karnes R. J., Bergstralh E. J., Davicioni E., Ghadessi M., Buerki C., Mitra A. P., Crisan A., Erho N., Vergara I. A., Lam L. L., Carlson R., Thompson D. J., Haddad Z., Zimmermann B., Sierocinski T., Triche T. J., Kollmeyer T., Ballman K. V., Black P. C., Klee G. G., Jenkins R. B. (2013) Validation of a genomic classifier that predicts metastasis following radical prostatectomy in an at risk patient population. *J Urol.* 190:2047–53. doi:10.1016/j.juro.2013.06.017.

[36] Klein E. A., Haddad Z., Yousefi K., Lam L. L., Wang Q., Choeurng V., Palmer-Aronsten B., Buerki C., Davicioni E., Li J., Kattan M. W., Stephenson A. J., Magi-Galluzzi C. (2016) Decipher Genomic Classifier Measured on Prostate Biopsy Predicts Metastasis Risk. *Urology.* 90:148–52. doi: 10.1016/j.urology.2016.01.012.

[37] Klein E. A., Yousefi K., Haddad Z., Choeurng V., Buerki C., Stephenson A. J., Li J., Kattan M. W., Magi-Galluzzi C., Davicioni E. (2014) A genomic classifier improves prediction of metastatic disease within 5 years after surgery in node-negative high-risk prostate cancer patients managed by radical prostatectomy without adjuvant therapy. *Eur Urol.* 67:778–86. doi:10.1016/j.eururo.2014.10.036.

[38] Cooperberg M. R., Davicioni E., Crisan A., Jenkins R. B., Ghadessi M., Karnes R. J. (2015) Combined value of validated clinical and genomic risk stratification tools for predicting prostate cancer mortality in a high-risk prostatectomy cohort. *Eur Urol.* 67:326–33. doi:10.1016/j.eururo.2014.05.039.

[39] Lobo J. M., Dicker A. P., Buerki C., Davicioni E., Karnes R. J., Jenkins R. B., Patel N., Den R. B., Showalter T. N. (2015) Evaluating the clinical impact of a genomic classifier in prostate cancer using individualized decision analysis. *PLoS One.* 10, e0116866. doi:10.1371/journal.pone.0116866.

[40] Sommariva S., Tarricone R., Lazzeri M., Ricciardi W., Montorsi F. (2016) Prognostic Value of the Cell Cycle Progression Score in Patients With Prostate Cancer: A Systematic Review and Meta-Analysis. *Eur Urol.* 69(1):107–15. doi: 10.1016/j.eururo.2014.11.038.

[41] Cuzick J., Stone S., Fisher G., Yang Z. H., North B. V., Berney D. M., Beltran L., Greenberg D., Møller H., Reid J. E., Gutin A., Lanchbury J. S., Brawer M., Scardino P. (2015) Validation of an RNA Cell Cycle Progression Score for Predicting Death From Prostate Cancer in a Conservatively Managed Needle Biopsy Cohort. *Br J Cancer.* 113(3):382–9. doi: 10.1038/bjc.2015.223.

[42] Cuzick J., Swanson G. P., Fisher G., Brothman A. R., Berney D. M., Reid J. E., Mesher D., Speights V. O., Stankiewicz E., Foster C. S., Møller H., Scardino P., Warren J. D., Park J., Younus A., Flake D. D., Wagner S., Gutin A., Lanchbury J. S., Stone S. (2011) Prognostic Value of an RNA Expression Signature Derived From Cell Cycle Proliferation Genes in Patients With Prostate Cancer: A Retrospective Study. *Lancet Oncol.* 12(3):245–55. doi: 10.1016/S1470-2045(10)70295-3.

[43] Bishoff J. T., Freedland S. J., Gerber L., Tennstedt P., Reid J., Welbourn W., Graefen M., Sangale Z., Tikishvili E., Park J., Younus A., Gutin A., Lanchbury J. S., Sauter G., Brawer M., Stone S., Schlomm T. (2014) Prognostic Utility of the Cell Cycle Progression Score Generated From Biopsy in Men Treated With Prostatectomy. *J Urol.* 192(2):409–14. doi:10.1016/j.juro.2014.02.003.

[44] Cuzick J., Stone S., Fisher G., Yang Z. H., North B. V., Berney D. M., Beltran L., Greenberg D., Møller H., Reid J. E., Gutin A., Lanchbury J. S., Brawer M., Scardino P. (2015) Validation of an RNA Cell Cycle Progression Score for Predicting Death From Prostate Cancer in a Conservatively Managed Needle Biopsy Cohort. *Br J Cancer.* 113(3):382–9. doi: 10.1038/bjc.2015.223.

[45] "Understanding the Prolaris Report." (2021) In: *Myriad Prolaris.* Available at: https://prolaris.com/understanding-the-prolaris-report/ [Retrieved Feb 28,2021;.

[46] Shore N. D., Kella N., Moran B., Boczko J, Bianco F. J., Crawford E. D., Davis T., Roundy K. M., Rushton K., Grier C., Kaldate R., Brawer M. K., Gonzalgo M. L. (2016) Impact of the Cell Cycle Progression Test on Physician and Patient Treatment Selection for Localized Prostate Cancer. *J Urol.* 195(3):612–8. doi: 10.1016/j.juro.2015.09.072.

[47] de Pouvourville G. (2015) Cost-effectiveness analysis for the use of the CCP score in the management of early low-risk prostate cancer in the French context. *Value Health*. 18(7):A358. doi: 10.1016/j.jval.2015.09.680.

[48] Kornberg Z., Cooperberg M. R., Cowan J. E., Chan J. M., Shinohara K., Simko J. P., Tenggara I., Carroll P. R. (2019) A 17-Gene Genomic Prostate Score as a Predictor of Adverse Pathology in Men on Active Surveillance. *J Urol*. 202(4):702-9. doi: 10.1097/JU.0000000000000290.

[49] Klein E. A., Cooperberg M., Magi-Galluzzi C., Simko J. P., Falzarano S. M., Maddala T., Chan J. M., Li J., Cowan J. E., Tsiatis A. C., Cherbavaz D. B., Pelham R. J., Tenggara-Hunter I., Baehner F. L., Knezevic D., Febbo P. G., Shak S., Kattan M. W., Lee M., Carroll P. R. (2014) A 17-gene assay to predict prostate cancer aggressiveness in the context of Gleason grade heterogeneity, tumor multifocality, and biopsy undersampling. *Eur Urol*. 66(3):550-60.

[50] doi: 10.1016/j.eururo.2014.05.004.

[51] Cullen J., Rosner I. L., Brand T. C., Zhang N., Tsiatis A. C., Moncur J., Ali A., Chen Y., Knezevic D., Maddala T., Lawrence H. J., Febbo P. G., Srivastava S., Sesterhenn I. A., McLeod D. G. (2014) A Biopsy-based 17-gene Genomic Prostate Score Predicts Recurrence After Radical Prostatectomy and Adverse Surgical Pathology in a Racially Diverse Population of Men with Clinically Low- and Intermediate-risk Prostate Cancer. *Eur Urol*. 68(1):123-31. doi: 10.1016/j.eururo.2014.11.030.

[52] Van Neste L., Bigley J., Toll A., Otto G., Clark J., Delrée P., Van Criekinge W., Epstein J. I. (2012) A Tissue Biopsy-Based Epigenetic Multiplex PCR Assay for Prostate Cancer Detection. *BMC Urol*. 12:16. doi: 10.1186/1471-2490-12-16.

[53] Heichman K. A., Warren J. D. (2012) DNA Methylation Biomarkers and Their Utility for Solid Cancer Diagnostics. *Clin Chem Lab Med*. 50(10):1707–21. doi: 10.1515/cclm-2011-0935.

[54] Trock B., Brotzman M., Mangold L., Bigley J. W., Epstein J. I., McLeod D., Klein E. A., Jones J. S., Wang S., McAskill T., Mehrotra J., Raghavan B., Partin A. W. (2012) Evaluation of GSTP1 and APC methylation as indicators for repeat biopsy in a high-risk cohort of men with negative initial prostate biopsies. *BJU Int*. 110:56-62.

[55] Partin A. W., Van Neste L., Klein E. A., Marks L. S., Gee J. R., Troyer D. A., Rieger-Christ K., Jones J. S., Magi-Galluzzi C., Mangold L. A., Trock B. J., Lance R. S., Bigley J. W., Van Criekinge W., Epstein J. I. (2014) Clinical validation of an epigenetic assay to predict negative histopathological results in repeat prostate biopsies. *J Urol*. 192:1081–7. doi:10.1016/j.juro. 2014.04.013.

[56] Van Neste L., Herman J. G., Otto G., Bigley J. W., Epstein J. I., Van Criekinge W. (2012) The epigenetic promise for prostate cancer diagnosis. *Prostate*. 1;72(11):1248–1261. doi:10.1002/pros.22459.

[57] Stewart G. D., Van Neste L., Delvenne P., Delrée P., Delga A., McNeill S. A., O'Donnell M., Clark J., Van Criekinge W., Bigley J., Harrison D. J. Clinical utility of an epigenetic assay to detect occult prostate cancer in histopathologically negative biopsies: results of the MATLOC study. *J Urol*. 2013;189:1110-1116. doi: 10.1016/j.juro.2012.08.219.

[58] Van Neste L., Partin A. W., Stewart G. D., Epstein J. I., Harrison D. J., Van Criekinge W. (2016) Risk Score Predicts High-Grade Prostate Cancer in DNA-methylation Positive, Histopathologically Negative Biopsies. *Prostate.* 76(12):1078–87. doi: 10.1002/pros.23191.

[59] Gurioli G., Martignano F., Salvi S., Costantini M., Gunelli R., Casadio V. (2018) GSTP1 methylation in cancer: a liquid biopsy biomarker? *Clin Chem Lab Med.* Apr 25;56(5):702-717. doi: 10.1515/cclm-2017-0703.

[60] Wojno K. J., Costa F. J., Cornell R. J., Small J. D., Pasin E., Van Criekinge W., Bigley J. W., Van Neste L. (2014) Reduced Rate of Repeated Prostate Biopsies Observed in ConfirmMDx Clinical Utility Field Study. *Am Health Drug Benefits.* 7(3):129–34.

[61] Wang W., Wang M., Wang L., Adams T. S., Tian Y., Xu J. (2014) Diagnostic ability of %p2PSA and prostate health index for aggressive prostate cancer: a meta-analysis. *Sci Rep.* May 23;4:5012. doi: 10.1038/srep05012.

[62] Alford A. V., Brito J. M., Yadav K. K., Yadav S. S., Tewari A. K., Renzulli J. (2017) The Use of Biomarkers in Prostate Cancer Screening and Treatment. *Rev Urol.* 19(4):221–34. doi: 10.3909/riu0772 .

[63] Shipitsin M., Small C., Choudhury S., Giladi E., Friedlander S., Nardone J., Hussain S., Hurley A. D., Ernst C., Huang Y. E., Chang H., Nifong T. P., Rimm D. L., Dunyak J., Loda M., Berman D. M., Blume-Jensen P. (2014) Identification of proteomic biomarkers predicting prostate cancer aggressiveness and lethality despite biopsy-sampling error. *Br J Cancer.* 111:1201–1212. doi: 10.1038/bjc.2014.396.

[64] Blume-Jensen P., Berman D. M., Rimm D. L., Shipitsin M., Putzi M., Nifong T. P., Small C., Choudhury S., Capela T., Coupal L., Ernst C., Hurley A., Kaprelyants A., Chang H., Giladi E., Nardone J., Dunyak J., Loda M., Klein E. A., Magi-Galluzzi C., Latour M., Epstein J. I., Kantoff P., Saad F. (2015). Biology of Human Tumors Development and clinical validation of an in situ biopsy-based multimarker assay for risk stratification in prostate cancer. *Clin Cancer Res.* 21(11):2591–2600. doi:10.1158/1078-0432.

[65] Saad F., Latour M., Lattouf J. B., Widmer H., Zorn K. C., Mes-Masson A. M., Ouellet V., Saad G., Prakash A., Choudhury S., Han G., Karakiewicz P., Richie J. P. (2017) Biopsy based proteomic assay predicts risk of biochemical recurrence after radical prostatectomy. *J Urol.* 197:1034–1040. Doi: 10.1016/j.juro.2016.09.116.

[66] Peabody J. W., DeMaria L. M., Tamondong-Lachica D., Florentino J, Czarina Acelajado M, Ouenes O, Richie J. P., Burgon T. (2017) Impact of a protein-based assay that predicts prostate cancer aggressiveness on urologists' recommendations for active treatment or active surveillance: a randomized clinical utility trial. *BMC Urol.* 17:51. doi: 10.1186/s12894-017-0243-1.

[67] Shariat S. F., Kattan M. W., Vickers A. J., Karakiewicz P. I., Scardino P. T. (2009) Critical review of prostate cancer predictive tools. *Future Oncol.* Dec;5(10):1555–84.

Chapter 8

Serum Markers of Prostate Cancer (A Review)

Maxim N. Peshkov[1,2,*]
and Igor V. Reshetov[1,2,†]

[1]Academy of postgraduate education under FSCC of FMBA of RUSSIA, Moscow, Russia
[2]FSAEI HE I.M. Sechenov First MSMU MOH Russia (Sechenovskiy University), Moscow, Russia

Abstract

Prostate cancer is one of the most frequent tumours in the world. The use of the prostate-specific antigen biomarker PSA for screening, diagnosis, and prognosis has resulted in advances in diagnosing and treating this disease. The PSA test's low cancer specificity necessitates the hunt for new potential patterns.

Because of the capabilities of current molecular genetic technologies, blood serum is an ideal diagnostic medium for disease detection and prognosis. Modern molecular genetic technologies allow for detecting genetic, epigenetic, and post-genomic alterations. A blood sample or liquid biopsy may enable systematic genomic evolution tracking and provide insight into the genetic landscape of all cancer lesions, both primary and progressed. Tumor cells release free DNA (cfDNA), proteins, and peptides into the bloodstream. Comprehensive examination of human serum fluid, accessible and accurate, opens new avenues for identifying illness patterns and providing data for future research.

New biomarkers for prostate cancer have emerged recently. While some of these markers outperform primary screening, others (such as the K4Score) benefit cancer risk stratification, grade assessment, and adverse

---

[*] Corresponding Author's Email: drpeshkov@gmail.com.
[†] Corresponding Author's Email: reshetoviv@mail.ru.

In: A Closer Look at Cancer Biomarkers
Editor: Arli Aditya Parikesit
ISBN: 979-8-89113-497-3
© 2024 Nova Science Publishers, Inc.

event prediction. One of these markers, proPSA, which is part of the Prostate Health Index (PHI), has been cleared for clinical use by the FDA. However, clinical laboratories certified under the Clinical Laboratory Improvement Amendment (CLIA) bought additional FDA-approved markers.

This review looks at the analytical capabilities of new blood indicators for prostate cancer detection and prognosis.

Keywords: prostate cancer (PCa), serum markers, biomarkers, prostate-specific antigen (PSA), K4Score, microRNA, circulating tumour cells (CTCs)

1.0. Introduction

Prostate cancer (PCa) is a severe medical and social concern affecting men of socially active ages worldwide. It is the second most prevalent cause of cancer-related death in men and the fifth most significant cause worldwide [1].

In most circumstances, revealing the earlier condition would increase the chances of successful treatment or reasonable control, which can considerably lessen the severity of the patient's impact on life or prevent or delay further consequences [2].

Due to a lack of particular biomarkers, late stages reveal more frequent discovery of diseases. As a result, early molecular diagnosis is critical for improving survival. Currently, the need for an easy-to-use and inexpensive sample technology and an accurate and portable platform for early disease detection are significant obstacles that seriously impede clinical diagnosis development [3].

Blood serum is a diagnostic fluid that comprises cells, nucleic acids, a significant number of proteins, and peptides; it is appealing because it offers numerous vital advantages for illness detection and prognosis, such as low cost and convenience of sample collection and processing [4].

A comprehensive investigation of human serum can help understand the pathophysiology and offer a foundation for identifying possible disease biomarkers [5].

Biomarkers are biomolecules linked to an elevated risk of disease and act as indicators of biological and pathological processes and physiological and pharmacological reactions to therapeutic therapy. Due to its clinical relevance, the identification of illness biomarkers in serum has considerable potential for personalized medicine, particularly for disease diagnosis and prognosis [6].

Identifying sensitive and specific biomarkers for early detection, prognostic assessment, and illness surveillance is a significant challenge in clinics. Proteome analysis utilizing human serum is a technological breakthrough that will allow the development of new biomarkers and biomarker patterns for various human disorders [7].

The rationale for choosing a biomarker in oncology is its ability to predict early detection, therapeutic response, and staging, as well as its ability to reduce the risk of overdiagnosis, differentiate between lesion types (to identify subclasses of prostate cancer), select different treatment options for patients, increase life expectancy, and provide a better quality of life. The most common classification for a biomarker is its application. Screening or early detection biomarkers can predict disease progression in men with asymptomatic cancer. Prognostic biomarkers predict disease progression in patients with probable cancer, whereas diagnostic biomarkers predict disease progression in patients with suspected cancer. In a subgroup of a patient population, prognostic biomarkers can indicate the probability of disease onset/progression or response to a specific medication. Finally, the utilization of surrogate biomarkers to replace a clinical endpoint and assess clinical benefit, harm, or absence of benefit or harm to the patient.

Numerous molecular biomarkers for prostate cancer are available; however, only a few are approved by the Food and Drug Administration (FDA) (PSA in 1994, phi in 2012, PCA3 in 2012) (Table 1).

Table 1. Serum biomarkers of prostate cancer

Biomarker	Molecular markers	Available as
Prostate Serum Antigen (tPSA)	PSA	FDA
PHI (Beckman Coulter Inc., Brea, CA, USA)	Total PSA, fPSA, p2PSA	FDA
K4Score (OPKO lab, Miami, FL, USA)	Total PSA, fPSA, intact PSA, hK2	CLIA-approved

2.0. Prostate-Specific Antigen and Its Derivatives

PSA is a 33 kDa serine protease encoded by the kallikrein 3 (KLK3) gene on chromosome 19q 13.3-13.4. Prostate epithelial cells release the PSA and have the primary purpose of liquefying sperm via proteolysis. This glycoprotein is typically found in low amounts in blood samples from healthy people [8].

1960 Flocks RH and colleagues were the first to detect antigens specific to human prostate tissue [9].

M. Hara et al. [10] of Japan's Scientific Center for Forensic Medicine described -selenoprotein, a human sperm antigen that, as found subsequently, matches PSA, in 1966. R. Ablin and colleagues proposed the recognized name PSA for the protein in 1970 when they were studying the antigenic characteristics of normal, benign, and cancerous pancreatic tissue [11].

PSA discovery is one of the twentieth century's great discoveries. The approval of the PSA test by the FDA in 1986 to track the progression of prostate cancer in diagnosed men. In 1994, the FDA approved the serum PSA test and digital rectal examination (DRE) for clinic-based prostate cancer screening [12].

Adenocarcinoma is distinguishable from benign inflammatory disease of the prostate gland by qualitative and quantitative changes in serum PSA levels. For example, protease inhibitors such as -1-antichymotrypsin (PSA-ACT) with 65% to 95% of total PSA (tPSA) are related; however, free PSA (fPSA) is the molecular form of PSA that does not occur in a protein complex. Although a low fPSA/tPSA ratio is a feature of prostate cancer, differences in the stability of molecular forms of PSA warn against using PSA as the primary screening approach in the clinic [13].

Benign prostatic hyperplasia (BPH), an inflammation known as prostatitis, raises PSA levels in the blood serum, resulting in needless biopsies [14]. As a result, there is agreement on the benefits of PSA-based prostate cancer screening. The decision to regularly check people aged 55-69 should be customized, and patients aged 70 years and older should refrain from undertaking this test. Men should be able to discuss the potential benefits and drawbacks of PSA testing with their healthcare professional and weigh their values and preferences before deciding to undertake screening" [15].

2.2. Prostate Health Index (PHI)

The Prostate Health Index (PHI) could detect clinically relevant prostate cancer. Free PSA is a collection of isoforms that do not have enzymatic activity and do not form complexes, including immature PSA, proPSA, and benign PSA (BPSA). ProPSA has three variants, each retaining all or part of the seven amino acid sequence. - [2] ProPSA is a peptide precursor of mature PSA generated preferentially in cancer cells [16].

An immunohistochemical study of prostate cancer tissues using monoclonal antibodies revealed that among the three isoforms, [-2] proPSA is most linked with cancer cells [17].

Two mathematical formulas defined two new clinical factors to improve the clinical usage of [-2]proPSA:

- ([p2PSA/10]/fPSA) - p2PSA%
- ([-2] proPSA / fPSA $\sqrt{PSA}$) - Prostate Health Index (PHI). Beckman Coulter Hybritech.

Based on the histological evaluation, the Prostate Health Index (phi; Beckman Coulter, Brea, California, USA) is a blood test that analyses fPSA, tPSA, and [-2]proPSA (p2PSA) levels to predict the likelihood of having an aggressive tumour (Gleason 7) [18].

The advantage of utilizing PHI in the clinic is that it reduces the number of needless biopsies obtained from individuals with borderline PSA levels while still detecting aggressive tumours.

The FDA approved the phi test 2012 to differentiate prostate cancer from other benign illnesses in males over 50 with regular digital rectal examination (DRE) results and serum tPSA levels ranging from 4 to 10 ng/mL. Using phi improves the specificity or diagnosis of prostate cancer in males with PSA levels ranging from 4 to 10 ng/ml. A score of 27.0 predicted prostate cancer on biopsy with a sensitivity of 90% and specificity of 31.1% [19].

A meta-analysis of 16 published studies [20] testing phi for identifying high-grade prostate cancer (Gleason score 7) revealed a pooled sensitivity of 0.90 and a pooled specificity of 0.17 (AUC 0.67 for high-grade malignancy). A recent multicenter trial of 658 men with PSA levels ranging from 4 to 10 ng/mL found that phi was superior to free and total PSA in detecting prostate cancer and improved clinically relevant high-grade prostate cancer prediction. Based on Epstein criteria, phi had a higher AUC (0.698) than %fPSA (0.654), p2PSA (0.550), and PSA (0.549) for clinically significant prostate cancer [17].

Using the PHI test in conjunction with multiparametric magnetic resonance imaging (mpMRI) aids in determining the requirement for a repeat biopsy. It improves the detection of clinically significant PCa [21]. The PHI test results have an impact on patients' clinical management. A low PHI level delays biopsy, but a high PHI level indicates an intermediate/high probability of having PCa with a high risk of progression [22].

The cost-effectiveness of incorporating PHI into the decision-making process for the requirement for a prostate biopsy has been validated [23].

Another potential application of the PHI test is the prediction of BCR following RP [24].

The National Comprehensive Cancer Network (NCCN) guidelines for 2023 endorsed the use of phi for early identification of prostate cancer but not as a first-line screening for all patients due to "limited prospective analyses in US populations." According to the panel, a PHI score greater than 35 indicates the chance of prostate cancer. It is "potentially informative for patients who have never undergone a biopsy or have had a negative biopsy" [25].

3.0. K4Score

The 4Kscore test (OPKO Health, Inc. Miami, Florida, USA) is a mathematical method (Figure 1) that determines the likelihood of clinically severe prostate cancer (Gleason score 7). This test assesses four kallikrein protein indicators (total PSA, free PSA, intact PSA, and human kallikrein-related peptidase 2) as well as other clinical data (age, digital rectal examination findings, and prior biopsy results) [26, 27]. Men with a low 4Kscore can safely postpone biopsy (Table 2).

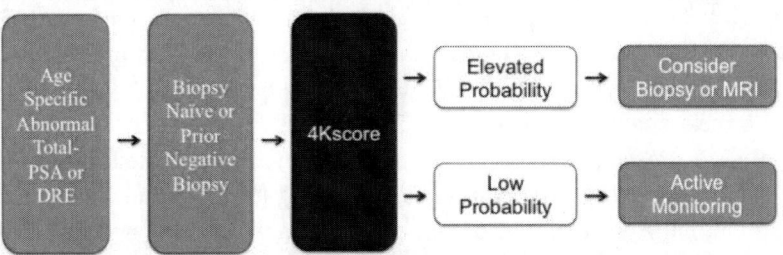

Figure 1. Algorithm for using the K4Score test.

Table 2. Reference intervals for 4Kscore test results

Risk of developing an aggressive tumour type	K4Score test value
Low	< 7,5
Medium	7,5 – 19,5
High	≥ 20,0

D.J. Parekh and colleagues examined the outcomes of patients who had a prostate biopsy [28]. Diagnostic performance of the 4Kscore test for clinically relevant prostate cancer (ROC AUC - 0.82). The 4Kscore test algorithm offers predictive ability for the risk of metastasis [29]. These findings imply that a 4Kscore test is appropriate to add crucial information to the clinical decision-making process for men with an abnormal PSA level or digital rectal examination result considering an initial or repeat prostate biopsy. The high-risk 4Kscore test result could identify men at high risk of aggressive prostate cancer who would benefit from a prostate biopsy to avoid the adverse and potentially deadly outcomes of prostate cancer [30].

In predicting high-grade prostate cancer, a direct comparison of K4score and Phi revealed equal improvement in discrimination [27]. The 4Kscore test is now available in a variety of nations throughout the world. The 4Kscore test is unnecessary as a second-line study in professional society clinical recommendations. The rationale for use is to establish the importance of performing a prostate gland puncture biopsy to confirm the diagnosis [26].

4.0. Micro-RNA

Since their discovery in 1993, miRNAs have emerged as a novel class of short RNAs that play an essential role in gene expression regulation. MicroRNAs (or miRs) are endogenous short (18-25 nucleotide) non-coding RNAs that regulate post-transcriptional gene expression by base complementarity between the miRNA's source area and the target mRNA's 3' untranslated region (UTR) [31]. MiRNAs bind to complementary regions in messenger RNAs (mRNAs) to limit translation or induce cleavage of specific target mRNAs [32].

Because post-transcriptional control of gene expression by microRNAs is critical, microRNAs can affect almost 60% of all human protein-coding genes [33]. Because of their role in gene expression, microRNAs have recently been dubbed "master regulators of gene expression" [34]. MiRNAs play a crucial role in carcinogenesis by beginning and promoting progression [35].

Over 4800 mature human microRNAs are currently known and registered in miRBase v22 (http://www.mirbase.org). MicroRNAs are strong indicators due to their propensity to remain stable in plasma and serum [36].

Table 3 shows a human miRNA dataset (tissue miRNA expression levels) retrieved from The Cancer Genome Atlas (TGCA), the most comprehensive repository of molecular and clinical data on human cancer. When microRNAs are associated with primary prostate cancer, signature sets with diagnostic

(Table 3) and prognostic (Table 4) features for prostate cancer can be discovered.

Table 3. Analytical capabilities of miRNAs in prostate cancer
(CI = confidence interval; PC = prostate cancer; N = normal sample)

Parameter	mi RNA Diagnostic Signature	Accuracy	AUC
PC vs. N 52 vs 52	Let-7a/b/c/i, miR-15b, miR-17, miR-20a, miR-21, miR-24, miR-25, miR-26a/b, miR-31, miR-32, miR-34b, miR-93, miR-106a, miR-141, miR-143, miR-145, miR-148a, miR-155, miR-182, miR-187, miR-200b, miR-218, miR-221, miR-223, miR-375	97.18% +/- 4.31% (CI 95%): 96.35–98.00	0.989 +/- 0.016 (CI 95%): 98.59–99.20

The accuracy and AUC of 29-miRNA in diagnosing patients with PCa vs. normal samples are high in Table 3, indicating that this miRNA profile may be a trustworthy tool for identifying patients with PCa from healthy controls in the same independent research set data.

Accuracy and area under the curve (AUC) for seven miRNA prognostic markers in Table 4. CI stands for confidence interval.

Table 4. Prognostic characteristics of miRNAs in prostate cancer.
(CI = confidence interval; PC = prostate cancer; N = normal sample)

Classification	Seven miRNA Prognostic Signature	Accuracy	AUC
P1 + P2 vs. P5 138 vs. 138	let-7a, miR-141, miR-145, miR-195, miR-221, miR-375, miR-451	71.38% (CI 95%): 70.79–71.96	74.7% (CI 95%): 73.28–76.11
P3 + P4 vs. P5 138 vs. 138	let-7a, miR-141, miR-145, miR-195, miR-221, miR-375, miR-451	61.59% (CI 95%): 60.71–62.46	61.6% (CI 95%): 60.24–62.95
P1 + P2 vs. P3 + P4 164 vs. 164	let-7a, miR-141, miR-145, miR-195, miR-221, miR-375, miR-451	65.26% (CI 95%): 64.51–66.00	66.8% (CI 95%): 66.10–67.49

In the different TCGA datasets studied, seven miRNAs with predictive ability performed poorly (Table 4). Indeed, as demonstrated in Table 4, the accuracy and AUC of the 7-miRNA signature in PCa prognosis are low for P1 + P2 versus P5 (71.38% and 74.7%, respectively), P3 + P4 versus P5 [37.% and 61.6%, respectively), and L1+L2 versus L3+L4 (65.26% and 66.8%, respectively) [37]. Given the new risk classification for patients with PCa, a greater understanding of their relevance as prognostic indicators is required [38].

Several criteria should produce the best noninvasive microRNA-based bodily fluid diagnostics for PCa diagnosis in the future. The standardization of extracellular miRNA purification techniques is one challenge. Because miRNA profiling is a multistep process (blood collection, plasma or serum isolation, RNA purification, RNA quantification, quality control, and RNA profiling), each stage may have methodological concerns and potential hazards [39]. As a result, considerable work has established common and standardized methods for best practice. Another problem when studying extracellular miRNAs is data normalization [40].

The use of liquid biopsy in screening to identify early instances is promising, and it opens up the possibility of providing personalized medication swiftly and in real time. MiRNAs are appealing targets for screening, diagnosis, prognosis, tumour progression tracking, biomarker discovery, and guiding correct patient treatment. Because they regulate the expression of specific target genes, such as tumour suppressors and oncogenes, their dysregulation changes in various molecular processes in tissues, contributing to some malignancies' complexity and heterogeneity. MiRNA studies rely on tissue samples or bodily fluids because miRNAs are exceptionally durable in serum, plasma, and urine, making them particularly appealing for noninvasive examinations.

Finally, future studies on deploying such innovative devices will consider the primary benefits for the early identification of prostate cancer, among other things. Furthermore, this molecular support will result in a more holistic approach to therapeutic strategies.

5.0. Circulating Tumor Cells (CTCs)

The term "liquid biopsy" refers to one of the most popular areas of molecular oncology. The core of this approach is to identify and monitor tumour-specific indicators (single altered cells, nucleic acids, proteins) in various body fluids (blood, urine, pleural fluid, and others). Current "liquid biopsy" occurrences are used in circumstances of early diagnosis, tumour persistence, or recurrence.

In 1969, Thomas Ashworth revealed the existence of epithelial cells in a dying cancer patient. He proposed that these were tumour cells, potentially explaining the presence of many tumour metastases in the patient at distinct anatomical places [41].

CTCs in peripheral blood from primary tumours or metastatic locations circulate through blood arteries and spread throughout the body [42].

When performing a liquid biopsy, examine the following parameters accordingly:

Investigate the following parameters during a liquid biopsy: - CTC is a pool of malignant cells that quickly separate from the tumour and stay in the bloodstream. In many malignant neoplasms, their discovery indicates hematogenous spread, corresponding with overall and relapse-free survival [43].

ctDNA and ctRNA are components of the extracellular pool of circulating nucleic acids found in human blood, which consumes massive molecular genetic information regarding secretion [44]. The carcinogenesis of breast, colon, prostate, and other malignancies has been removed [45].

Exosomes are membrane vesicles whose role in intercellular communication is due to the transfer of functional biomolecules (microRNA, lipids, carbohydrates, low molecular weight compounds), thereby potentiating various aspects of carcinogenesis: modification of the microenvironment, increased tumour cell invasiveness, the presence of angiogenesis, tuning drug heredity functions, activation of oncogenic and anti-apoptotic signalling pathways, suppression of antitumor immunity, and others. [46].

Early detection of CTCs may aid doctors in identifying more aggressive tumours that may benefit from a program of careful surveillance and more intensive therapy when clinical recurrence occurs. They play a role in cancer metastasis, and CTC protein expression and localization at the cellular level were very diverse, reflecting both the source tumour and the site of metastasis [46].

CellSearch technology is now the only FDA-approved test for early diagnosis of metastatic PCa, playing an essential role in castration-resistant tumours due to PSA's lack of sensitivity and specificity at this stage. Because PSA testing lacks sensitivity and specificity in patients with metastatic castration-resistant prostate cancer (mCRPC), CTCs are an intriguing marker that may lead to early diagnosis of castration-resistant status, allowing clinicians to achieve more individualized treatment planning, controlled tumour response, and treatment progression. With these prospective applications, CTC detection and identification is a promising technology that could solve several issues connected with the clinical detection and treatment of PCa [47].

Thalgott et al. investigated the role of CTCs in the early stages of prostate cancer using CellSearch in patients with high-risk, locally progressed, metastasis-resistant, and taxane-resistant PCa (Table 5). According to the findings of this study, the number of CTCs in patients with taxane-refractory metastases was considerably higher than in patients with high-risk locally progressed illness. Furthermore, patients with bone and visceral involvement had higher mean CTC counts than controls, whereas patients with soft tissue metastases had CTC counts equivalent to controls. CTC counts correlated positively with serum alkaline phosphatase and LDH levels but negatively with haemoglobin and PSA doubling time [48]. Combining the findings of this research indicates a limit in CTCs' diagnostic relevance in the early stages of the disease.

Table 5. Analytical capabilities of CellSearch technology in prostate cancer

CTCs detected in patients with metastatic prostate cancer:
- ⩾2 CTCs in 57% of metastatic PCa blood samples, 14% of which contained ⩾50 CTCs, whereas these were extremely rare in healthy subjects [49].
- Independent correlation between CTCs blood concentration detected by CellSearch system and OS [50].
- No correlation between CTC levels and response to treatment [51].
CTC, circulating tumor cell; OS, overall survival; PCa, prostate cancer.

It is interesting to note that in PCa, CTC detection plays a crucial role, mainly in the later stages of the disease. Indeed, unlike kidney and bladder cancer, early-stage PCa can be treated with PSA, a validated and sensitive soluble biomarker used to detect and monitor disease before castration occurs. Resistant state. For this reason, CTC assessment evaluated advanced stages, with particular interest in its prognostic role and response prediction.

Conclusion

The gold standard for identifying prostate cancer is the histological assessment of prostate tissue collected using transrectal ultrasound-guided needle biopsy (TRUS). The Gleason score [52] is the most often used scale for determining the stage of prostate cancer. The higher the Gleason score, the more likely the cancer will spread quickly [53].

Furthermore, the European Randomised Prostate Cancer Screening Trial discovered that when PSA utilized the PCa screening method alone, about

50% of patients were overdiagnosed [54]. Screening patients for PCa is still debatable and not recommended due to the risk of overtreatment [55].

Despite advancements in prostate cancer treatment, increased PSA levels and abnormal digital rectal examination (DRE; nodular, indurated, and asymmetry) still necessitate referral for investigation [56]. The second most prevalent finding that merits further examination for malignancy is abnormal DRE [57]. As a result, many patients with increased PSA/abnormal DRE are transferred to secondary care when invasive and costly treatments are performed [58]. It was frequently unneeded because over 75% of individuals referred for additional examination have a negative biopsy [59].

Furthermore, 2.5-3% of patients come to the hospital within a week of the TRUS treatment with a significant infection (urinary tract infection and bacterial prostatitis). Better decision-making in primary care could prevent this, but clinicians should retrieve more biological information about the patient's disease. No biomarkers or biomarker combinations with sensitivity and specificity for PSA substitution have been found [60].

As a result, improved ways to distinguish individuals with prostate disease who require treatment or surveillance from those who do not. Symptoms and PSA levels are not reliable indicators of the disease. Indeed, no PSA result is fully diagnostic [61], as a patient with a PSA >10 ng/mL may not have cancer, but another patient with a PSA 1 ng/mL may have an aggressive disease. As a result, there is an urgent need for novel tests that can, at the very least, stratify individuals and, ideally, be diagnostic. However, given the varied nature of PCa, a single biomarker is unlikely to be diagnostic.

This review highlights new molecular biomarkers for prostate cancer that are beginning to play a vital role in improving diagnosis and treatment. The good news is that there is already a promising collection of biomarkers; nonetheless, clinicians and reimbursement agencies have a significant challenge: evaluating and prioritizing new indicators.

These indicators can assist doctors in determining the need for biopsy, particularly in individuals with grey zone PSA values ranging from 4.0 to 10.0 ng/mL, avoiding unnecessary biopsies. These biomarkers may also help differentiate clinically relevant prostate cancer and guide treatment regimens. Liquid biopsy, multi-omics, sophisticated imaging, and technology integration are also in the works. Clinically verified robust biomarkers, in conjunction with an integrated imaging method such as multiparametric magnetic resonance imaging (MRI), can enable more individualized risk assessment for prostate cancer diagnosis and therapy.

The available and expanding body of literature and pace of prostate cancer biomarker research, as well as the development of highly integrated supercomputing platforms, will likely lead to more exciting discoveries that will improve individualized risk assessment and clinical management of the disease. Multicenter research financed by biotech/pharmaceutical businesses and government bodies such as The National Cancer Institute (NCI) Early Detection Research Network (EDRN) will continue to provide much-needed advice and resources for these advancements.

Effective prostate cancer treatment requires a precise diagnosis. The clinician's issue is distinguishing benign conditions (BGE) from PCa, which has comparable symptoms. PSA testing has a negative benefit-harm ratio in population estimates [62]. Thus, biomarkers contributing to PSA sensitivity and specificity may provide additional information to clinicians, allowing them to make a more informed management decision about referring the patient to secondary care for further testing or to refer the patient to primary care.

Additional Information

Financing the work. Review and analytical work on the manuscript preparation carried out at the personal expense of the author.

Conflict of interest. The author declares that there are no apparent or potential conflicts of interest related to the publication of this article.

Authors' participation: collection, analysis of literature data, writing the article - Peshkov M.N., editing the article - Reshetov I.V.

All authors read and approved the final version of the manuscript before publication.

References

[1] Bray F., Ferlay J., Soerjomataram I., Siegel R. L., Torre L. A., Jemal A. Global cancer statistics 2018: Globocan estimates of incidence and mortality worldwide for 36 cancers in 185 countries. *Cancer J. Clin.* 2018;68:394–424. doi: 10.3322/caac.21492.

[2] Gutiérrez-Sánchez, G., Atwood, J., Kolli, V. S., Roussos, S., Augur, C. (2012). Initial proteome analysis of caffeine-induced proteins in Aspergillus tamarii using

two-dimensional fluorescence difference gel electrophoresis. *Applied Biochemistry and Biotechnology*, 166(8), 2064–77.

[3] Schwenk, J., Harmel, N., Zolles, G., Bildl, W., Kulik, A., Heimrich, B., Chisaka, O., Jonas, P., Schulte, U., Fakler, B., Klöcker, N. (2009). Functional proteomics identify cornichon proteins as auxiliary subunits of AMPA receptors. *Science*, 323(5919), 1313–9.

[4] Marondedze, C., Thomas, L. A. (2012). Apple hypanthium firmness: new insights from comparative proteomics. *Applied Biochemistry and Biotechnology*, 168(2), 306–26.

[5] Yu, C., Xu, C., Xu, L., Yu, J., Miao, M., Li, Y. (2012). Serum proteomic analysis revealed diagnostic value of haemoglobin for nonalcoholic fatty liver disease. *Journal of Hepatology*, 56(1),241–7.

[6] Zhang A., Sun H., Sun W., Ye Y., Wang X. (2013). Proteomic identification network analysis of haptoglobin as a key regulator associated with liver fibrosis. *Applied Biochemistry and Biotechnology*, 169(3), 832–46.

[7] Arbing, M. A., Kaufmann, M., Phan, T., Chan, S., Cascio, D., Eisenberg, D. (2010). The crystal structure of the *Mycobacterium tuberculosis* Rv3019c-Rv3020c ESX complex reveals a domain-swapped heterotetramer. *Protein Science*, 19(9), 1692–703.

[8] Balk S. P., Ko Y.-J., Bubley G. J. Biology of prostate-specific antigen. *J. Clin. Oncol.* 2003;21:383–391. doi:10.1200/JCO.2003.02.083.

[9] Flocks R. H., Bandhaur K., Patel C., Begley B. J. Studies on Sperma- agglutinating antibodies in antihuman prostate sera. *J Urol*. 1962;87(3):475-478. https://doi.org/10.1016/S0022-5347(17)64982-6.

[10] Hara M., Inoue T., Koyanagi Y., Gotoh J., Yamazaki H., Fukuyama T. Preparation and immunoelectrophoretic assessment of antisera to human seminal plasma. *Nippon Hoigaku Zasshi*. 1966;20:356. (Abstract in Japanese).

[11] Ablin R. J., Bronson P., Soanes W. A., Witebsky E. Tissue - and species-specific antigens of normal human prostatic tissue. *J Immu- nol*. 1970;104(6):1329-1339.

[12] Catalona W. J., Smith D. S., Ratliff T. L., Dodds K. M., Coplen D. E., Yuan J. J., Petros J. A., Andriole G. L. Measurement of prostate-specific antigen in serum as a screening test for prostate cancer. *N. Engl. J. Med.* 1991;324:1156–1161. doi: 10.1056/NEJM199104253241702.

[13] Khan M. A., Sokoll L. J., Chan D. W., Mangold L. A., Mohr P., Mikolajczyk S. D., Linton H. J., Evans C. L., Rittenhouse H. G., Partin A. W. Clinical utility of propsa and "benign" psa when percent free psa is less than 15%. *Urology*. 2004;64:1160–1164. doi: 10.1016/j.urology.2004.06.033.

[14] Vickers A. J., Cronin A. M., Aus G., Pihl C. G., Becker C., Pettersson K., Scardino P. T., Hugosson J., Lilja H. A panel of kallikrein markers can reduce unnecessary biopsy for prostate cancer: Data from the European randomized study of prostate cancer screening in Goteborg, Sweden. *BMC Med*. 2008;6:19. doi: 10.1186/1741-7015-6-19.

[15] Bibbins-Domingo K., Grossman D. C., Curry S. J. The US Preventive Services Task Force 2017 draft recommendation statement on screening for prostate cancer: An invitation to review and comment. *JAMA*. 2017 doi: 10.1001/jama.2017.4413.

[16] Chan T. Y., Mikolajczyk S. D., Lecksell K., Shue M. J., Rittenhouse H. G., Partin A. W., Epstein J. I. Immunohistochemical staining of prostate cancer with monoclonal antibodies to the precursor of prostate-specific antigen. *Urology.* 2003;62:177–181. doi: 10.1016/S0090-4295(03)00138-9.

[17] Loeb, S.; Catalona, W. J. The Prostate Health Index: A new test for the detection of prostate cancer. *Ther. Adv. Urol.*, 2014, 6(2), 74-77.

[18] Siegel R. L., Miller K. D., Jemal A. Cancer statistics, 2019. *Cancer J. Clin.* 2019;69:7–34. doi: 10.3322/caac.21551; 27.

[19] Catalona W. J., Partin A. W., Sanda M. G., Wei J. T., Klee G. G., Bangma C. H., Slawin K. M., Marks L. S., Loeb S., Broyles D. L., Shin S. S., Cruz A. B., Chan D. W., Sokoll L. J., Roberts W. L., van Schaik R. H., Mizrahi I. A. A multicenter study of [−2]pro-prostate specific antigen combined with prostate specific antigen and free prostate specific antigen for prostate cancer detection in the 2.0 to 10.0 ng/ml prostate specific antigen range. *J. Urol.* 2011;185:1650–1655. doi: 10.1016/j.juro.2010.12.032.

[20] Wang W., Wang M., Wang L., Adams T. S., Tian Y., Xu J. Diagnostic ability of %p2psa and prostate health index for aggressive prostate cancer: A meta-analysis. *Sci. Rep.* 2014;4:5012. doi: 10.1038/srep05012.

[21] Druskin S. C., Tosoian J. J., Young A., Collica S., Srivastava A., Ghabili K., Macura K. J., Carter H. B., Partin A. W., Sokoll L. J., Ross A. E., Pavlovich C. P. Combining Prostate Health Index density, magnetic resonance imaging and prior negative biopsy status to improve the detection of clinically significant prostate cancer. *BJU Int.* 2018;121:619–626. doi: 10.1111/bju.14098.

[22] White J., Shenoy B. V., Tutrone R. F., Karsh L. I., Saltzstein D. R., Harmon W. J., Broyles D. L., Roddy T. E., Lofaro L. R., Paoli C. J., Denham D., Reynolds M. A. Clinical utility of the Prostate Health Index (phi) for biopsy decision management in a large group urology practice setting. *Prostate Cancer Prostatic Dis.* 2018;21:78–84. doi: 10.1038/s41391-017-0008-7.

[23] Huang D., Wu Y., Lin X., Xu D., Na R., Xu J. Cost-Effectiveness Analysis of Prostate Health Index in Decision Making for Initial Prostate Biopsy. *Front. Oncol.* 2020;10:565382. doi: 10.3389/fonc.2020.565382.

[24] Lughezzani G., Lazzeri M., Buffi N. M., Abrate A., Mistretta F. A., Hurle R., Pasini L., Castaldo L., De Zorzi S. Z., Peschechera R., Fiorini G., Taverna G., Casale P., Guazzoni G. Preoperative prostate health index is an independent predictor of early biochemical recurrence after radical prostatectomy: Results from a prospective single-center study. *Urol. Oncol.* 2015;33:337.e7–337.e14. doi: 10.1016/j.urolonc.2015.05.007.

[25] Kelvin A. M., Preston C. S., Bahler C., Box G., Carlsson S. V., Catalona W. J., Dahl D. M., Dall'Era M., Davis J. W., Drake B. F., Epstein J. I., Etzioni R. B., Farrington T. A., Garraway I. P., Jarrard D., Kauffman E., Kaye D., Kibel A. S., LaGrange C. A., Maroni P., Ponsky L., Reys B., Salami S. S., Sanchez A., Seibert T. M., Shaneyfelt T. M., Smaldone M. C., Sonn G., Tyson M. D., Vapiwala N., Wake R., Washington S., Yu A., Yuh B., Berardi R. A., Freedman-Cass D. A. NCCN Guidelines® Insights: Prostate Cancer Early Detection, Version 1.2023. *J Natl Compr Canc Netw.* 2023 Mar;21(3):236-246. doi: 10.6004/jnccn.2023.0014.

[26] Bryant R. J., Sjoberg D. D., Vickers A. J. Predicting high-grade cancer at tecore prostate biopsy using four kallikrein markers measured in blood in the ProtecT study. *J Natl Cancer Inst* 2015;107(7):51-62.

[27] Nordstrom T., Vickers A., Assel M. Comparison between the four-kallikrein panel and prostate health index for predicting prostate cancer. *Eur Urol* 2015; 68(1):139-46.

[28] Parekh D. J., Punnen S., Sjoberg D. D., Asroff S. W., Bailen J. L., Cochran J. S., Concepcion R., David R. D., Deck K. B., Dumbadze I., Gambla M., Grable M. S., Henderson R. J., Karsh L., Krisch E. B., Langford T. D., Lin D. W., McGee S. M., Munoz J. J., Pieczonka C. M., Rieger-Christ K., Saltzstein D. R., Scott J. W., Shore N. D., Sieber P. R., Waldmann T. M., Wolk F. N., Zappala S. M. A multi-institutional prospective trial in the USA confirms that the 4Kscore accurately identifies men with high-grade prostate cancer. *Eur Urol*. 2015;68(3):464–70. doi:10.1016/j.eururo.2014.10.021.

[29] Pär Stattin., Andrew J. Vickers., Daniel D Sjoberg., Robert Johansson., Torvald Granfors., Mattias Johansson., Kim Pettersson., Peter T. Scardino., Göran Hallmans., Hans Lilja. Improving the Specificity of Screening for Lethal Prostate Cancer Using Prostate-specific Antigen and a Panel of Kallikrein Markers: A Nested Case-Control Study. *Eur Urol*. 2015 Aug;68(2):207-13. doi: 10.1016/j.eururo. 2015.01.009.

[30] Daniel D. Sjoberg., Andrew J. Vickers., Melissa Assel., Anders Dahlin., Bing Ying Poon., David Ulmert., Hans Lilja. Twenty-year Risk of Prostate Cancer Death by Midlife Prostate-specific Antigen and a Panel of Four Kallikrein Markers in a Large Population-based Cohort of Healthy Men. *Eur Urol*. 2018 Jun;73(6):941-948. doi: 10.1016/j.eururo.2018.02.016.

[31] Lee R. C., Feinbaum R. L., Ambros V. The C. elegans heterochronic gene lin-4 encodes small RNAs with antisense complementarity to lin-14. *Cell*. (1993) 75:843–54. 10.1016/0092-8674(93)90529-y.

[32] Bartel D. P. MicroRNAs: genomics, biogenesis, mechanism, and function. *Cell*. 2004;116(2):281–97.

[33] Friedman R. C., Farh K. K-H., Burge C. B., Bartel D. P. Most mammalian mRNAs are conserved targets of microRNAs. *Genome Res*. (2009) 19:92–105. 10.1101/gr.082701.108.

[34] Garofalo M., Croce C. M. microRNAs: master regulators as potential therapeutics in cancer. *Annu Rev Pharmacol Toxicol*. (2011) 51:25–43. 10.1146/annurev-pharmtox-010510-100517.

[35] Croce C. M. Causes and consequences of microRNA dysregulation in cancer. *Nat Rev Genet*. 2009;10(10):704–14. doi:10.1038/nrg2634.

[36] Mitchell P. S., Parkin R. K., Kroh E. M., Fritz B. R., Wyman S. K., Pogosova-Agadjanyan E. L., Peterson A., Noteboom J., O'briant K. C., Allen A., Lin D. W., Urban N., Drescher C. W., Knudsen B. S., Stirewalt D. L., Gentleman R., Vessella R. L., Nelson P. S., Martin D. B., Tewari M. Circulating microRNAs as stable blood-based markers for cancer detection. *Proc. Natl. Acad. Sci. USA*. 2008;105:10513–10518. doi: 10.1073/pnas.0804549105.

[37] Martens-Uzunova E. S., Jalava S. E., Dits N. F., van Leenders G. J., Moller S., Trapman J., Bangma C. H., Litman T., Visakorpi T., Jenster G. Diagnostic and prognostic signatures from the small non-coding RNA transcriptome in prostate cancer. *Oncogene.* 2012;31:978–991. doi: 10.1038/onc.2011.304.

[38] Loeb S., Montorsi F., Catto J. W. Future-proofing Gleason grading: What to call Gleason 6 prostate cancer? *Eur. Urol.* 2015;68:1–2. doi: 10.1016/j.eururo.2015.02.038.

[39] Moldovan L., Batte K. E., Trgovcich J., Wisler J., Marsh C. B., Piper M. Methodological challenges in utilizing miRNAs as circulating biomarkers. *J. Cell. Mol. Med.* 2014;18:371–390. doi: 10.1111/jcmm.12236.

[40] Weber J. A., Baxter D. H., Zhang S., Huang D. Y., Huang K. H., Lee M. J., Galas D. J., Wang K. The microRNA spectrum in 12 body fluids. *Clin. Chem.* 2010;56:1733–1741. doi: 10.1373/clinchem.2010.147405.

[41] Ashworth T., "A case of cancer in which cells similar to those in the tumours were seen in the blood after death" *Australasian Medical Journal*, vol. 14, no. 3, pp. 146–149, 1869.

[42] Riquet, M., C. Rivera., L. Gibaultetal. Lymphatic spread of lung cancer: Anatomical lymph node chains unchained in zones. *Revue de Pneumologie Clinique*, vol. 70, no. 1-2, pp. 16–25, 2014.

[43] Jia S., Zhang R., Li Z., Li J. Clinical and biological significance of circulating tumor cells, circulating tumor DNA, and exosomes as biomarkers in colorectal cancer. *Oncotarget.* 2017 Apr 18; 8 (33):55632–55645. doi: 10.18632/oncotarget.17184.

[44] Arneth B. Update on the types and usage of liquid biopsies in the clinical setting: a systematic review. *BMC Cancer.* 2018 May 4; 18 (1):527. doi: 10.1186/s12885-018-4433-3.

[45] Tai Y. L., Chen K. C., Hsieh J. T., Shen T. L. Exosomes in cancer development and clinical applications. *Cancer Sci.* 2018 Aug; 109 (8): 2364–2374. doi: 10.1111/cas.13697.

[46] Fidler, I. J. "The pathogenesis of cancer metastasis: the seed and soil hypothesis revisited." *Nature Reviews Cancer*, vol. 3, no. 6, pp. 453–458, 2003.

[47] Ciccarese C., Montironi R., Fiorentino M., Martignoni G., Brunelli M., Iacovelli R., Lopez Beltran A., Cheng L., Scarpelli M., Much H., Tortora G., Massari F. Circulating tumor cells: a reliable biomarker for prostate cancer treatment assessment? *Curr Drug Meta.* Epub ahead of print May 18, 2017. doi: 10.2174/1389200218666170518163549.

[48] Thalgott M., Rack B., Maurer T., Souvatzoglou M., Eiber M., Kreß V., Heck M. M., Andergassen U., Nawroth R., Gschwend J. E., Retz M. Detection of circulating tumor cells in different stages of prostate cancer. *J Cancer Res Clin Oncol* 2013; 139: 755–763.

[49] de Bono J. S., Scher H. I., Montgomery R. B., Parker C., Miller M. C., Tissing H., Doyle G. V., Terstappen L. W., Pienta K. J., Raghavan D. Circulating tumor cells predict survival benefits from treatment in metastatic castration-resistant prostate cancer. *Clin Cancer Res* 2008; 14: 6302–6309.

[50] Fleisher M., Danila D. C., Fizazi K., Hirmand M., Selby B., de Bono S. P., Scher H. Circulating tumor cell (CTC) enumeration in men with metastatic castration-

resistant prostate cancer (mCRPC) treated with enzalutamide post-chemotherapy (phase 3 AFFIRM study). *J Clin Oncol* 2015; (Suppl.): abstract 5035;.

[51] Stott S. L., Lee R. J., Nagrath S., Yu M., Miyamoto D. T., Ulkus L., Inserra E. J., Ulman M., Springer S., Nakamura Z., Moore A. L., Tsukrov D. I., Kempner M. E., Dahl D. M., Wu C. L., Iafrate A. J., Smith M. R., Tompkins R. G., Sequist L. V., Toner M., Haber D. A., Maheswaran S. Isolation and characterization of circulating tumor cells from patients with localized and metastatic prostate cancer. *Sci Transl Med* 2010; 2:25ra23.

[52] Rubin M. A., Dunn R., Kambham N., Misick C. P., O'Toole K. M. Should a Gleason Score be Assigned to a Minute Focus of Carcinoma on Prostate Biopsy? *Am J Surg Pathol* (2000) 24(12):1634–40. doi: 10.1097/00000478-200012000-00007.

[53] Epstein J. I. Prostate Cancer Grading: A Decade After the 2005 Modified System. *Mod Pathol* (2018) 31(S1):47–63. doi: 10.1038/modpathol.2017.133].

[54] Alberts A. R., Schoots I. G., Roobol M. J. Prostate-Specific Antigen-Based Prostate Cancer Screening: Past and Future. *Int J Urol* (2015) 22(6):524–32. doi: 10.1111/iju.

[55] Stark J. R., Mucci L., Rothman K. J., Adami H. O. Screening for Prostate Cancer Remains Controversial. *BMJ* (2009) b3601:339. doi: 10.1136/bmj.b3601;.

[56] Palmerola R., Smith P., Elliot V., Reese C. T., Mahon F. B., Harpster L. E., Icitovic N., Raman J. D. The Digital Rectal Examination (DRE) Remains Important-Outcomes From a Contemporary Cohort of Men Undergoing an Initial 12-18 Core Prostate Needle Biopsy. *Can J Urol* (2012) 19(6):6542–7.

[57] Galosi A. B., Palagonia E., Scarcella S., Cimadamore A., Lacetera V., Delle Fave R. F., Antezza A., Dell'Atti L. Detection Limits of Significant Prostate Cancer Using Multiparametric MR and Digital Rectal Examination in Men With Low Serum PSA: Up-Date of the Italian Society of Integrated Diagnostic in Urology. *Arch Ital Di Urol E Androl* (2021) 93(1):92–100. doi: 10.4081/aiua.2021.1.92.

[58] Young S. M., Bansal P., Vella E. T., Finelli A., Levitt C., Loblaw A. Guideline for Referral of Patients With Suspected Prostate Cancer by Family Physicians and Other Primary Care Providers. *Can Fam Physician* (2015) 61(1):33–9.

[59] Prostate Cancer Diagnosis and Management Guidance NICE. Available at: https://www.nice.org.uk/guidance/ng131/chapter/Recommendations#assessment-and-diagnosis.

[60] Mcnally C. J., Ruddock M. W., Moore T., Mckenna D. J. Biomarkers That Differentiate Benign Prostatic Hyperplasia From Prostate Cancer: A Literature Review. *Cancer Manag Res* (2020) 12:5225–41. doi: 10.2147/CMAR.S250829.

[61] Duffy M. J. Biomarkers for Prostate Cancer: Prostate-Specific Antigen and Beyond. *Clin Chem Lab Med* (2020) 58(3):326–39. doi: 10.1515/cclm-2019-0693.

[62] Alberts A. R., Schoots I. G., Roobol M. J. Prostate-Specific Antigen-Based Prostate Cancer Screening: Past and Future. *Int J Urol* (2015) 22(6):524–32. doi: 10.1111/iju.12750.

About the Editor

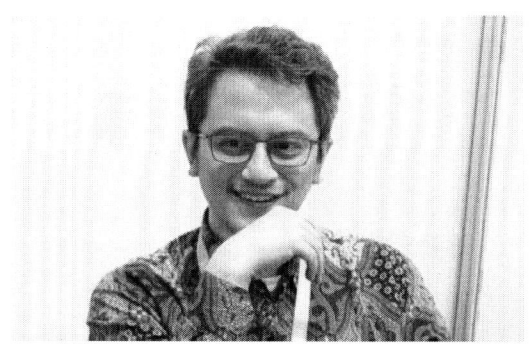

Arli Aditya Parikesit
Department of Bioinformatics, School of Life Sciences, Indonesia International Institute for Life Sciences

Arli Aditya Parikesit is a scientist who specializes in bioinformatics, the field that combines biology, computer science, and mathematics. He is currently the Vice-Rector of Research and Innovation at the Indonesia International Institute for Life Sciences (I3L), where he also teaches as a faculty member of the Bioinformatics Department. He obtained his bachelor's and master's degrees in Chemistry from the University of Indonesia, and then received a full scholarship from the German Academic Exchange Service (DAAD) to pursue his doctoral degree in Bioinformatics at the University of Leipzig, Germany. His doctoral research focused on using modern techniques to annotate protein domains for the three domains of life. He is also an expert in immunoinformatics, in-silico drug design, and in-silico transcriptomics. He has published many papers in international journals and received several awards and grants for his research. He is also a member of the Indonesian Young Academy of Science (ALMI) and the Indonesian Chemical Society. He is passionate about advancing the science and technology of bioinformatics in Indonesia and beyond.

Email: arli@daad-alumni.de.

Index

A

analysis, 3, 5, 6, 9, 10, 11, 12, 13, 16, 19, 26, 31, 33, 34, 40, 41, 44, 49, 53, 55, 56, 59, 60, 64, 65, 66, 67, 68, 72, 76, 79, 81, 83, 87, 89, 94, 95, 102, 104, 106, 107, 108, 109, 111, 114, 115, 116, 117, 118, 121, 123, 131, 132, 133
antibody, 11, 14, 22, 48
antigen, 8, 9, 11, 14, 19, 22, 23, 24, 39, 40, 69, 79, 81, 86, 101, 121, 122, 133, 134

B

binding, 10, 11, 13, 14, 17, 19, 20, 21, 22, 23, 24, 29, 30, 31, 32, 33, 34, 35, 36, 37, 38, 59, 83
bioinformatics, xi, xiii, 1, 2, 3, 4, 5, 6, 7, 8, 9, 54, 55, 56, 67, 137
biological, 2, 34, 37, 54, 55, 59, 65, 67, 71, 72, 75, 76, 79, 81, 82, 86, 102, 120, 130, 135
biomarker(s), ix, xi, xii, xiii, 3, 5, 6, 39, 40, 41, 42, 43, 44, 45, 46, 47, 48, 49, 51, 69, 70, 71, 72, 74, 75, 76, 78, 79, 80, 81, 82, 83, 84, 86, 87, 88, 89, 91, 92, 93, 94, 95, 96, 99, 110, 111, 114, 117, 118, 119, 120, 121, 127, 129, 130, 131,135, 136
body fluids, 43, 49, 71, 72, 75, 88, 99, 127, 135
BPIFA1, 8, 9, 10, 11, 14, 22, 24

C

carcinogenesis, xi, 1, 42, 89, 94, 99, 125, 128

central nerve system (CNS), 53, 54
circulating extracellular DNA, 70
circulating tumour cells (CTCs), 44, 45, 50, 76, 120, 127, 128, 129
ConfirmMDx®, 91, 92
construct, 8, 11, 12, 14, 15, 16, 22, 23, 24

D

Decipher®, 91, 92
diagnosis, ix, xi, xii, 3, 6, 37, 38, 39, 40, 41, 44, 45, 49, 69, 70, 72, 73, 74, 75, 78, 80, 82, 85, 86, 89, 91, 92, 95, 96, 117, 119, 120, 121, 123, 125, 127, 128, 130, 131, 136
docking, 13, 19, 20, 21, 24, 27, 29, 31, 34, 36, 37, 38
domain, 31, 32, 34, 36, 38, 108, 132
drug target, 30, 34

E

epitopes, 8, 9, 10, 11, 14, 15, 16, 19, 20, 21, 22, 23, 24, 25, 26

G

gene markers, 53, 65, 66
genetic expression, 1, 3
genetic(s), 1, 3, 4, 5, 37, 39, 40, 41, 44, 46, 48, 57, 58, 70, 76, 77, 85, 91, 92, 94, 97, 98, 99, 101, 102, 103, 107, 110, 112, 113, 119, 128

H

herbal, 32, 33, 34, 35
heterogeneity, 49, 76, 78, 83, 85, 92, 93, 94, 95, 96, 99, 106, 110, 112, 113, 114, 117, 127
HLA, 8, 10, 11, 13, 14, 17, 18, 19, 20, 21, 22, 24

I

Indonesia, xii, xiii, 1, 5, 7, 8, 10, 11, 13, 14, 15, 24, 25, 29, 36, 53, 55, 66, 137

K

K4Score, 119, 120, 121, 124

M

medulloblastoma, 53, 54, 55, 56, 61, 62, 63, 65, 66, 67, 68
metabolic, 81, 82, 86
metabolites, 32, 33, 71, 80, 81, 82, 83, 87
metabolomic(s), 70, 81, 82, 86, 87, 88, 89
microarrays, 3, 5, 54, 58, 59, 67, 101
microRNA, 41, 70, 73, 88, 89, 115, 120, 127, 128, 134, 135
molecular docking, xii, 13, 19, 20, 21, 24, 27, 29, 30, 31, 32, 34, 36, 37, 38
molecular genetic markers, 92
multiplex analysis of urine markers, 70

N

natural compound, 29, 30, 32, 33, 34, 35, 36, 37, 38
non-small cell lung cancer (NSCLC), xi, 7, 8, 9, 22, 24, 25, 26, 27, 44, 45, 49, 50, 87, 88, 89

O

Oncotype Dx®, 92
origin, 72, 73

P

peptide, 7, 9, 10, 11, 12, 13, 15, 17, 22, 24, 25, 26, 122
population, xi, 7, 8, 9, 10, 11, 13, 14, 15, 22, 24, 43, 50, 62, 85, 97, 98, 115, 117, 121, 131, 134
precision medicine, 40, 51, 73, 87, 112
prevention, xii, 25, 27, 37, 40, 42, 49, 75, 92
Prolaris®, 91, 92
Promark®, 91, 92, 112
prostate cancer (PCa), xii, 29, 30, 31, 33, 36, 37, 38, 39, 40, 41, 42, 49, 69, 70, 71, 72, 73, 76, 77, 78, 79, 80, 81, 82, 83, 84, 85, 86, 87, 88, 89, 91, 92, 93, 94, 95, 96, 97, 98, 99, 100, 101, 102, 103, 104, 105, 106, 107, 108, 109, 110, 112, 113, 114, 115, 116, 117, 118, 119, 120, 121, 122, 123, 124, 125, 126, 127, 128, 129, 130, 131, 132, 133, 134, 135, 136
prostate tumours, 70, 71, 95
prostate-specific antigen (PSA), 49, 69, 70, 72, 78, 79, 80, 81, 83, 84, 85, 91, 92, 93, 96, 101, 105, 107, 109, 113, 119, 120, 121, 122, 123, 124, 125, 128, 129, 130, 131, 132, 133, 136
protein, 1, 2, 3, 4, 5, 6, 9, 11, 12, 22, 24, 26, 27, 30, 31, 34, 35, 36, 37, 38, 40, 41, 44, 45, 58, 67, 71, 77, 78, 82, 96, 110, 111, 118, 122, 124, 125, 128, 132, 137
proteomic, xi, 81, 112, 118, 132

R

ribosomal protein, 53, 65, 66
risk prediction, 92
RNA marker, 70

S

screening, 3, 29, 31, 39, 40, 41, 42, 43, 49, 51, 69, 70, 71, 88, 89, 118, 119, 121, 122, 124, 127, 129, 132, 134, 136
serum markers, 120

structural bioinformatics, xi, 1, 2, 3, 5
support vector machine, 26, 53, 60, 67

T

targeted therapy, 8, 40, 41, 46, 47, 50
tissue biomarker, 75, 91, 92, 94, 95, 96, 112
transcription factors, 30, 31, 32, 33, 34, 35, 36, 37
treatment, ix, xi, xii, 4, 6, 7, 8, 22, 25, 30, 31, 33, 37, 38, 39, 40, 41, 43, 44, 45, 46, 47, 48, 49, 50, 51, 56, 61, 66, 67, 70, 71, 72, 73, 74, 75, 76, 84, 86, 91, 94, 95, 96, 98, 99, 103, 104, 105, 107, 112, 116, 118, 120, 121, 127, 128, 129, 130, 131, 135
tumor, xi, 1, 46, 54, 67, 77, 80, 87, 117, 119, 127, 129, 135, 136

U

urine, xi, 42, 43, 69, 70, 71, 72, 73, 74, 75, 76, 77, 78, 79, 80, 81, 82, 83, 84, 85, 86, 87, 88, 89, 96, 99, 101, 127

V

vaccine, xi, 7, 8, 9, 11, 12, 13, 14, 15, 16, 17, 22, 23, 24, 25, 26, 27
vector machine, 53, 56, 60, 67, 68